# FAST FACTS FOR DEVELOPING A NURSING ACADEMIC PORTFOLIO

## What You Really Need to Know in a Nutshell

D1564023

**Ruth A. Wittmann-Price, PhD, RN, CNS, CNE,** is the department chair and professor of nursing at Francis Marion University in Florence, SC. Ruth has been a perinatal nurse for 33 years. She received her AAS and BSN degrees from Felician College in Lodi, NJ (1978, 1981) and her MS as a Perinatal CNS from Columbia University, NY (1983). Ruth completed her PhD at Widener University, Chester, PA (2006), and was awarded the Dean's Award for Excellence. She developed a mid-range nursing theory "Emancipated Decision Making in Women's Health Care" and has tested her theory in three research studies. Other nurse researchers are now using her theory to test other decision-making situations in women's health care. Besides continuing her research about decisional science, she studies developmental outcomes of preterm infants.

Ruth has taught all levels of nursing students over the past 15 years and has completed an international service-learning trip. Ruth is co-editor of and chapter contributor to several books, including *Nursing Education: Foundations for Practice Excellence* (2007, F. A. Davis), which was an AJN Book of the Year Award winner; *Certified Nurse Educator (CNE) Review Manual* (2009, Springer Publishing Company); *NCLEX-RN® EXCEL: Test Success: An Unfolding Case Study Review* (2010, Springer Publishing Company); and *Maternal-Child Nursing Test Success Through Unfolding Case Study Review* (2011, Springer Publishing Company), an electronically enhanced print and e-book. Her chapters include "The Newborn at Risk" in *Maternal-Child Nursing Care: Optimizing Outcomes for Mothers, Children, and Families* (Ward, S., & Hinsley, S., Eds., 2009, F. A. Davis); and Wittmann-Price, R. A., Waite, R., & Woda, D. H., "The Role of the Educator" in *Role Development for Doctoral Advanced Nursing Practice* (Dreher, H. M., & Glasgow, M. E. S., Eds., 2011, Springer Publishing Company). She has published numerous articles and has presented her research regionally, nationally, and internationally.

# FAST FACTS FOR DEVELOPING A NURSING ACADEMIC PORTFOLIO

## What You Really Need to Know in a Nutshell

Ruth A. Wittmann-Price, PhD, RN, CNS, CNE

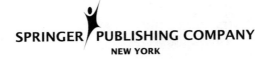

SPRINGER PUBLISHING COMPANY

NEW YORK

Springer Publishing Company, LLC
11 West 42nd Street
New York, NY 10036
www.springerpub.com

*Acquisitions Editor:* Margaret Zuccarini
*Composition:* Newgen Imaging

ISBN: 978-0-8261-2038-0
E-book ISBN: 978-0-8261-2039-7

11 12 13/ 5 4 3 2 1

The author and the publisher of this Work have made every effort to use sources believed
to be reliable to provide information that is accurate and compatible with the standards
generally accepted at the time of publication. The author and publisher shall not be liable
for any special, consequential, or exemplary damages resulting, in whole or in part, from
the readers' use of, or reliance on, the information contained in this book. The publisher
has no responsibility for the persistence or accuracy of URLs for external or third-party
Internet Web sites referred to in this publication and does not guarantee that any content
on such Web sites is, or will remain, accurate or appropriate.

**Library of Congress Cataloging-in-Publication Data**
Wittmann-Price, Ruth A.
  Fast facts for developing a nursing academic portfolio : what you really
need to know in a nutshell / Ruth A. Wittmann-Price.
     p. ; cm.
  Includes bibliographical references and index.
  ISBN 978-0-8261-2038-0 — ISBN 978-0-8261-2039-7 (e-book)
  I. Title.
  [DNLM: 1.  Faculty, Nursing—Handbooks. 2. Teaching—Handbooks.
3. Achievement—Handbooks. 4. Documentation—methods—Handbooks. 5. Job
Application—Handbooks. WY 49]
  650.14'2—dc23                                              2011040229

Printed in the United States of America by Hamilton Printing

# Contents

### Part III: Examples

# Exemplar Contributors

**Rhonda Brogdon, MSN, MBA, DNP, RN**
Assistant Professor, Nursing
Francis Marion University
Florence, South Carolina

**Frances H. Cornelius, MSN, PhD, RN-BC, CNE**
Associate Clinical Professor
Chair of the MSN Advanced Practice Role Department
Coordinator of Informatics Projects
Drexel University, College of Nursing and Health
    Professions Nursing Faculty
Philadelphia, Pennsylvania

**Jeana N. Dunn, BSN, RN**
Graduate of Francis Marion University (2010)
Staff RN, Maternal Child Health Services/
    Labor and Delivery
Florence, South Carolina

**Rosemary Fliszar, PhD, RN, CNE**
Certified Nurse Educator, Assistant Professor
Kutztown University
Bethlehem, Pennsylvania

**Karen K. Gittings, DNP, RN, CCRN**
Assistant Professor of Nursing
Francis Marion University
Florence, South Carolina

**Roberta Waite, EdD, APRN, CNS-BC**
Associate Professor of Nursing
and
Assistant Dean of Academic Integration and
   Evaluation of Community Programs
Drexel University
Philadelphia, Pennsylvania

# Foreword

Portfolios are collections of products and evidence that demonstrate your achievements. Nurses can develop a portfolio to document their clinical expertise, experiences in clinical practice, and professional goals. Similarly with academic portfolios, nursing faculty members can provide evidence of their research and scholarship, teaching performance, and contributions to the nursing program and profession. With a well-developed academic portfolio, nurse educators can document their accomplishments in relation to criteria for appointment and reappointment, promotion, tenure, merit review, and other purposes. Academic portfolios also are a strategy for educators to reflect on their development as a nursing faculty member, identify their strengths and weaknesses, and plan future activities to meet their career goals.

Few nurse educators are prepared to develop an academic portfolio: This book fills that gap. Beginning chapters explain the purposes of a portfolio and its value in assessing one's own professional growth, documenting achievements, and setting career goals. Later chapters explain how to develop a personal statement, describe teaching successes with evidence to support those achievements, document research and scholarship, and explain one's contributions to service and the nursing profession. Details on formatting and presenting an academic portfolio including how to develop an e-portfolio also are included in the book. Many times portfolios are developed to document performance, recognition, and impact as part of the educator's application for promotion and tenure; two chapters in the book explain how to gear a portfolio to those purposes.

Academic portfolios are important not only because they provide a means of documenting accomplishments in the faculty role but also because they enable an educator to reflect on his or her own progress in meeting career goals. With an academic portfolio, nursing faculty members can monitor their career development and present their work for others to review and critique. This is an easy-to-read book that will serve as a valuable resource for nursing faculty members in developing their academic portfolios.

*Marilyn H. Oermann, PhD, RN, FAAN, ANEF*
*Professor and Chair of Adult and Geriatric Health*
*School of Nursing*
*University of North Carolina at Chapel Hill*
*Editor,* Journal of Nursing Care Quality

# Preface

All nurse educators know that moving from clinical practice to academia includes culture shock! This book is designed for nurse educators who are considering entering academia or contemplating career advancement within academia. It is designed to discuss the importance of and specifics about developing an effective academic portfolio. How you, the novice or expert nurse educator, present yourself and your accomplishments through the presentation of an academic portfolio, is imperative to a successful career. Let's face it, academia differs greatly from our familiar practice settings. In order to accomplish your goal you must communicate clearly and effectively to the rest of the academic community about your scholarship. This book is designed to help you negotiate academia safely and effectively.

Formatting this book using the SBAR (Situation, Background, Assessment, and Recommendation) method of communication demonstrates the importance of telling your scholarly journey in a concise, explanatory manner with recommendations or reflections for further development in your role. In a clinical setting, SBAR is the communication tool that nurses use to provide other health care professionals the vital information needed about a patient. In this book it is used to communicate to nurses the vital information they need to know in order to present their accomplishments is a scholarly format. Scholarly presentation of nurse educators' work not only assists the individual but also assists the profession of nursing, which is a relatively young discipline, to be recognized for its excellent knowledge development.

I had been in several academic positions before I was exposed to a course designed to teach educators how to put together an academic portfolio. The course provided me with an experienced mentor, to whom I am grateful. The product that I developed after those learning sessions was more than I expected and considerably different from other evaluative material I had previously used. The product was reflective, thoughtful, and, most importantly, something that I could be proud of because it represented my best work and demonstrated to academic colleagues the nature of nursing scholarship!

I want to pass along that "something to be proud of feeling" to my colleagues by sharing with you in this book the information that was afforded to me and assisted me in my career. My portfolio not only assists me to gain professional advancement but it also influences my growth. There is something very therapeutic about putting together your professional achievements and goals in one place. It allows you to see "face-to-face" what you have done, where you need to go, and what directions need to be tweaked. It is a method to reflect on the strengths and limitations of your career in order to help you formulate new goals and ideals.

This book is arranged to walk you through the process of academic portfolio development step by step. But before that happens, the first section provides you with the background you need in order to understand the climate in which your professional evaluation will take place. Chapter 1 or "the situation" describes why an academic portfolio is so important for career advancement. The background in Chapter 2 provides a brief historical view of academic portfolio development. The third chapter is the assessment and may be the most important chapter. It explains variables in the academic environment that may affect the development of your academic portfolio. And the final chapter of the first part makes recommendations for the development of your portfolio.

Part II of this book provides the reader with the step by-step process in Chapters 5 through 9 that is needed to develop an academic portfolio. It provides explanations, Fast Facts in a Nutshell, and examples! Chapter 10 discusses the actual physical presentation of your material and provides great anecdotal gems in order to enhance your academic portfolio presentation. Chapter 11, by Dr. Frances H. Cornelius, describes the process for e-portfolio development, which is being used at some institutions.

The last two chapters of this book are actual academic portfolio personal statements in their entirety from two successful nursing academics. One nurse educator is from a smaller school; the other is from a larger university. This provides the readers with a comparison perspective. Each personal statement presented in Chapters 12 and 13 includes a critique to assist in explaining what the content in that specific section brings to the finished product. Finally, you will want to read about the contributors and their careers in order to better understand the context under which they offered their personal statements to benefit other nurse educators.

Nurse educators will enjoy this book and use it as a guide to develop their own amazing academic portfolios. Every academic portfolio will be different and every nurse educator will reflect upon it differently, but there are critical elements that all should contain. Developing these elements in such a way that they showcase you and nursing is very gratifying and will assist you to put your best foot forward in the academic setting!

*Ruth A. Wittmann-Price*

# Acknowledgments

I am thankful for my mentor of my first academic portfolio, Dr. Pamela A. Geller, Drexel University. Her patience, wisdom, and empathy guided me through the process and taught me a tremendous amount about presenting myself. I am deeply grateful.

I am also grateful to my Deans at Drexel University, Dr. Donnelley and Dr. Glasgow, for their continuing support in my career and for promoting academic excellence.

Thank you to the contributors of this book who gave so freely of themselves to help me complete the project and shared a piece of themselves with other nurse educators.

To my husband, David, and my children, Rachel, Samuel, and Rosemary, who are always supportive of my career—thank you. Finally, I would like to thank my two big sisters, Judy McDowell and Eileen Wittmann, who are my living guardian angels.

# FAST FACTS FOR DEVELOPING A NURSING ACADEMIC PORTFOLIO

## What You Really Need to Know in a Nutshell

# Using SBAR to Create Academic Portfolios for Nurse Educators

## Recommendations for Achieving Effective Academic Advancement

# Situation

## Why You Need to Develop Your Academic Portfolio!

### INTRODUCTION

*Nurse educators are entering academia at unprecedented numbers due to the call for a BSN-prepared workforce. Nurse educators, like you, are unique academics because most come to academia from the practice setting. The transition from practice to academia presents challenges, and nurse educators need the right tools to ensure success. One of the most important tools is a well-put-together academic portfolio to showcase your accomplishments. Academic portfolios are important not only during periods of career mobility; they also serve as a reflective mechanism that can assist you to gain insight into your career goals. Furthermore, academic portfolios can help other academics who may be unfamiliar with the profession of nursing to learn the scholarship that is unique to your practiced discipline. Although a resume or curriculum vitae (CV) may suffice in the practice realm as a representation of your*

> *work, a different format is needed in order to thoroughly demonstrate your accomplishments in academia. This is well explained by Luk, Yukawa, and Emery (2009): "The traditional CV does not adequately reflect the breadth and quality of a clinician-educator's work. The educator's portfolio is an alternative to the CV to accomplish this goal" (p. 497). This chapter will review the background information that will convince you to start your academic portfolio as soon as possible!*

At the end of this chapter, the nurse educator will be able to:

1. Identify reasons for developing your academic portfolio.
2. Discuss the areas of scholarship on which an academic portfolio will focus.
3. Understand the role of the nurse educator compared to other academics and your colleagues in practice settings.

Nurse educators must showcase their accomplishments or scholarship in the academic environment, yet most are not educated or mentored on the best method to do so. The development of an academic portfolio is a tool that you, the nurse educator, needs to assist you to succeed in academe. Academic portfolios serve three distinct but related purposes:

- Academic portfolios showcase your accomplishments and excellence in scholarship when you are:

  1. Interviewing for a job in academia
  2. Pursuing a promotion in academia
  3. Applying for tenure in academia

- When used as an ongoing developmental process tool, academic portfolios serve as an instrument to promote individual professional growth through the process of reflection.

- Academic portfolios teach other academics about the scholarship of nursing by developing a clear, concise, yet detailed professional presentation that adequately explains discipline-specific information.

*FAST FACTS in a NUTSHELL*

All three purposes are equally important to ensure a successful academic career and the nurse educator can incorporate all three into the single process of academic portfolio development.

To begin to understand the process of academic portfolio development, you should ask yourself three questions:

1. Have I recently taken a good, thoughtful look at where I was when I started my career, where I am now, and where I want to be?
2. What are my best academic accomplishments?
3. Do academic educators from other departments, who contribute to the search or interview, promotion, or tenure committees, understand the complex discipline of nursing?

## DEFINITIONS AND TYPES OF ACADEMIC PORTFOLIOS

An academic portfolio has been clearly defined as "...a visual representation of the individual, their experience, strengths, abilities, and skills" (McCready, 2007, p. 144), or "an autobiography of personal growth" (Javinen & Kohenen, 1995, p. 29). Oermann (2002) describes two types of portfolios: best work and growth and development

(p. 73). In actuality, academic portfolio development is an ongoing process. It should be started as soon as possible, reflectively evaluated often and revised, and the final product used for submission to show your best work for career change or advancement. Academic portfolios are a well-selected collection of reflections and evidence that show how you are developing personally and professionally (Casey & Egan, 2010). Academic portfolios serve as a logical solution to the multifaceted evaluative process needed for educators. They can be crafted to adequately represent you, your accomplishments, discipline, and scholarship.

## SCHOLARSHIP

Academic portfolios showcase accomplishments in the form of scholarship. Scholarship is defined as "learning; knowledge acquired by study" (Dictionary.com, 2011). It is the knowledge that a nurse educator gains and applies to outcomes within the role (Billings & Kowalski, 2008). It can take multiple forms such as finding a new innovative teaching technique, doing a pilot study to determine if students who are peer-tutored will increase test scores, presenting, or writing an article for a journal. Remember, "Scholarship demands rigor" (Martsolf, Dieckman, Cartechine, et al., 1999, p. 326). Good scholarship takes work, benefits our students, and promotes nursing knowledge.

Nurse educators are indeed scholars and this is best defined by Billings & Kowalski (2008) as "A *scholar* is a person who has particular knowledge in an area of specialization. A scholar has a spirit of inquiry and is able to think logically and communicate effectively" (p. 204). Therefore scholarship is something in which you are involved in on a day-to-day basis in academe. Many academic institutions will recognize and

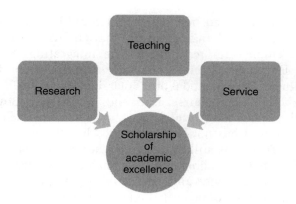

**FIGURE 1.1** Three areas of evaluation for academic educators.

organize scholarship as three distinct performance areas: research, teaching, and service. In traditional academic environments, an educator's performance will be evaluated in each area. Figure 1.1 gives a graphic depiction of model of scholarship.

## BOYER'S VIEW OF SCHOLARSHIP

There are other models of scholarship besides the traditional model of teaching, research, and service. One of the more popular alternative models is that of Boyer. In 1990, Ernest Boyer wrote a book entitled *Scholarship Reconsidered* that was well received by nurse educators. Boyer expanded on the three traditional categories of scholarship and added a fourth category. The categories that Boyer defined are discovery, integration, application, and teaching. Teaching is a key component in Boyer's model and is described as a transmitter of knowledge that links the other forms of scholarship (Boyer, 1990, p. 24).

Boyer demonstrated how his model could be adequately used in today's changing educational environment. The model emphasizes teaching as the integrating thread. Table 1.1 provides definitions and examples of the four domains of Boyer's model of scholarship.

Although many nurse academics agree with Boyer's model of scholarship, and some schools use it as the evaluation tool, it has not been embraced by all institutions. Many institutions still evaluate educators with the traditional models of scholarship that include only teaching, research, and service and, therefore, it is imperative you know how you will be evaluated and by what model.

---

**TABLE 1.1    Examples of Boyer's Model of Scholarship**

| | |
|---|---|
| **Discovery**<br>(Research)<br><br>Example: Comparing technology usage of 2nd degree and pre-licensure students. | **Integration**<br>(Interdisciplinary collaboration or unique ways of knowledge development)<br><br>Example: Using music therapy to decrease student test anxiety |
| **Application**<br>(Taking learned knowledge and putting it into practice)<br>Example: Taking students abroad to better understand cultural concepts. | **Teaching**<br>(Facilitating learning)<br>Example: Using an active teaching strategy such as gaming to increase knowledge acquisition. |

*Source:* Adapted from Nibert, M. (n.d.). *Boyer's Model of Scholarship.* Retrieved from http://www.webs1.uidaho.edu/mkyte/ui_strategic_plan_implementation/resources/Boyer

═══════════════════════*FAST FACTS in a NUTSHELL*

Find out how you will be evaluated by *carefully* reading your faculty handbook.

## ACADEMIA TODAY

Academic portfolios are important because successful academic careers are currently being redefined within educational institutions and there is an increasing call for faculty accountability. That accountability is being emphasized more and more due to many socioeconomic factors that include:

- The high cost of education
- Institutional demands for excellence to stay competitive
- The need to find better methods to evaluate faculty (Martsolf et al., 1999).

Faculty are meeting and often exceeding this increased call for accountability by providing evidence of their excellence in scholarship. Academic portfolios are the mechanism to best showcase the skills and abilities of educators, as well as provide a description of an educator's philosophy and attitude.

## SOCIAL INFLUENCES ON NURSE EDUCATORS

This section will discuss some of the reasons that academic preparation for nurse educators is more important now than ever.

## The Institute of Medicine

The Institute of Medicine (IOM) has recommended that 80% of nurses be educated at the baccalaureate level by 2020 (IOM, 2010). This recommendation is supported by well-grounded evidence that nurses educated at the baccalaureate level decrease morbidity and mortality statistics for patients (Aiken, Clarke, Cheung, Sloane, & Silber, 2003). The IOM recommendation will increase the need for nurse educators to assume roles in collegiate settings. Although many nurse educators are already functioning in academic settings, others are bound to move into academia in response to the call to increase baccalaureate-prepared nurses and the movement entitled "BSN in 10 years" that has been initiated by the American Nurses Association (American Nurses Association [ANA], 2008).

*FAST FACTS in a NUTSHELL*

RN to BSN programs are predicted to grow and will need an increasing number of nurse educators at the collegiate level.

The IOM is also calling for seamless educational transitions between levels of nursing education. When these recommendations are actualized, there will be an increased need for nurse educators in academic settings. Nurse educators can show their accountability through their academic portfolio.

## Magnet®

Another social force that is affecting the profession of nursing is the American Nurses Credentialing Center

(ANCC) Magnet Recognition Program® (ANCC, 2011) for health care practice centers. The certification is currently held by only 5% of U.S. hospitals (CHOP, 2011) and is based on criteria of nursing excellence. New criteria that hospitals and health care centers must follow when submitting an application read as follow: "Organizations submitting application anytime after January 1, 2011 and before 2013 . . . 100% of nurse managers must have at least a baccalaureate degree in nursing at time of application" (ANCC, 2011, p. 1).

=== *FAST FACTS in a NUTSHELL*

Hospitals and outpatient centers anticipating application for Magnet® certification will be encouraging nurses to return to school, which will also increase the need for nurse educators to enter academia.

At this point in history, with all these social forces pushing nursing education toward the collegiate setting, it is difficult to imagine that effective presentation of nurse educators' scholarship will not be needed.

## Faculty Shortage

Currently nurse educators are in a choice position due to the lack of nursing faculty. The shortage of nurse educators is described by the American Association of Colleges of Nursing (AACN, 2010):

. . . a total of 880 faculty vacancies were identified in a survey of 556 nursing schools with baccalaureate and/or graduate programs across the country (70.3% response rate). Besides the vacancies, schools cited the need to create an additional 257 faculty positions to accommodate student demand. The data show a national nurse faculty vacancy rate of 6.9%. (p. 1)

This employment advantage is unlike most other academics at this point in time. Therefore, nurse educators have options and can truly reflect upon and choose a position in academia that best suits their scholarship and skills. Developing an academic portfolio can assist with this self-evaluation and reflection.

## THE IMPORTANCE FOR NURSE EDUCATORS TO DEVELOP AN ACADEMIC PORTFOLIO

Nursing is a relatively new discipline to academia and it is unique in a number of ways when compared to traditional disciplines. It is of paramount importance for nurses and evaluators to recognize, understand, and incorporate these differences into nurse educators' academic portfolios to best represent both themselves and the discipline. The obvious difference between nursing and other disciplines is that it is a practice profession, and thus much of the teaching occurs in the clinical setting as opposed to the classroom. The teaching that occurs in the clinical setting is so different than what is normally evaluated in the academic settings that it is usually NOT an aspect that is evaluated in real time. Unfortunately, rarely do members of the academic community who serve on interview, promotion, or tenure committees come to a clinical setting to see a nurse educator "in action."

### *FAST FACTS in a NUTSHELL*

The real-time evaluation of the scholarship of teaching for nurse educators is more often done in the academically familiar classroom setting versus the practice-familiar clinical setting.

A second difference between nursing and many other academic disciplines is its educational history. Nursing was originally taught in diploma schools that did not mimic the academic setting. Even today nursing is still taught in over 100 diploma schools as well as in technical and community colleges. These programs, in effect, may have historically "branded" nursing in the view of some academics as a technical skill rather than an academic discipline. This may produce subliminal fallout in the evaluation process of nurse educators. Evaluators on promotion and tenure committees may not hold the nursing educator's scholarship at the same level as other educators if they are not knowledgeable about it and view it as a lesser academic discipline.

Another consideration why nurse educators may be evaluated differently is the lack of the nursing profession's consensus on entry into practice. Fuzzy lines of delineation exist due to diploma, technical, and academic education units. Other problems in the academic evaluation of nurse educators may arise due to the newness of the discipline in some institutions and evaluators' lack of knowledge about the discipline, especially if nursing is not represented on the evaluative or other institutional committees.

Third, nursing, like education, has been a female-dominated profession. Other disciplines in academia have been male dominated for years. When applying the theoretical concepts of critical social theory and feminist theory, it is easy to imagine how the evaluation process in academia may not favor female-dominated professions. This is another good reason to have nursing represented on university committees.

Additionally, nurse educators often come to academic positions later in their careers than other traditional academics. Therefore, they have not "grown up" in the system like other academics and are many times less savvy about

*FAST FACTS in a NUTSHELL*

A well-developed academic portfolio will assist nurse educators to overcome many of the actual or perceived social barriers to career advancement in academia.

the political context of the system. This is substantiated by the facts listed in LaRocco, 2006 (pp. 1–2).

- The average age of the nurse educator holding a PhD is 54
- The average age of doctorally prepared nursing faculty in baccalaureate and graduate nursing programs holding the rank of professor is 57.3. Among associate professors, the average age is 55; among assistant professors, it is 51
- The average age at which nursing faculty members retire is 62.5
- Less than 7% of nursing doctoral students are younger than 35; the median age for all research doctorate awardees is 33
- The average time from enrollment to degree completion for nursing PhDs is 8.3 years; for all research doctorate awardees, it is 6.8 years

Many nurse educators start in their academic careers later in life because they are in practice first. This may work as a double-edged sword: The nurse educator comes to the academic position with more personal maturity, but many times knows only the culture of the practice environment, which is far different than that of academia. Some of the environmental or cultural differences that have been noted are:

- Academia is less reactive to situations
- Academia is more stable due to tenure so people have been in positions and power longer

- Nurse educators must change focus from patient-centered to student-centered even in the clinical teaching area
- Being assertive is not always valued

============================*FAST FACTS in a NUTSHELL*

Nurse educators many times start in academia at a disadvantage, but with the proper mentoring and professional development can use their experience to promote their own success.

A final reason why nursing education evaluation may differ from other disciplines (with the exception of education) is that there is an outcome examination. Programs of nursing, unlike traditional disciplines in academia, have a direct outcome measure: NCLEX-RN® success. This single entity can create a silo of focus for evaluative committee members. When examination pass-rate percentages are low, fingers immediately start pointing to teaching deficits, but when passing percentages are high those concerns disappear. All nurse educators know that NCLEX-RN® success is a multifaceted process that encompasses a multitude of variables, including but not limited to those listed in Exhibit 1.1. Therefore, the tone of an academic portfolio may differ when nurse educators are being evaluated in years of NCLEX-RN® success as opposed to years when NCLEX-RN® success is not up to expectations.

In lieu of all the various reasons that can indirectly affect a faculty evaluation, a well-put-together academic portfolio is a must for you and every nurse educator. There are increasing social reasons for nurse educators to become more adept at presenting themselves in the best light, and therefore positioning themselves in leadership positions throughout the governing organization. Other

**Exhibit 1.1**    A List of Factors That May Affect NCLEX-RN® Success for Educational Units

- Leadership effectiveness
- Newness of faculty
- Cohesiveness of faculty group
- Sequencing of courses
- Concepts of the curricula
- Learner group dynamics and characteristics
- Learner group qualifications
- Local competition
- Financial restraints of the academic unit
- Mission or philosophy of the educational unit or governing institution
- Administrative support from the governing institution
- Lack of practice partners
- Lack of staff development resources
- Lack of faculty education in graduate work specific to nursing education
- Lack of support staff
- Unrealistic prerequisites required by the governing institution

academics will not understand the scholarship of nursing unless we, the nurse educators, teach them.

## PREPARING NURSE EDUCATORS FOR ACADEMIA

Although graduate education in nursing has been at the collegiate level for many years, the education is many times concentrated knowledge in a specialty area, such as pediatrics, and scant discussion is devoted to the subject of academic success in which many graduates may eventually teach. Being a "good nurse" or even a "good teacher" may not be enough. Nurse educators need to understand the expectations of academia and that nursing is just as accountable as all other disciplines to those standards and criteria of evaluation. Developing an academic portfolio is often a part of new faculty development, yet its significance to the nurse educators' future needs to be underscored (Supplee & Gardner, 2002).

=== *FAST FACTS in a NUTSHELL*

Doctorate of Nursing Practice (DNP) degrees are currently the fasted growing degrees in the field of nursing.

Although the DNP degree was originally a terminal degree intended for practice, many DNP graduates (30%) are entering into academic positions. Although teaching was not the intent of the DNP degree, these graduates are sorely needed in collegiate settings. The best scenario would be to increase DNP graduates' knowledge of the academic environment and of scholarship presentation to ensure their success in the environment (Wittmann-Price, Waite, & Woda, 2011). In addition, the IOM (2010) is also calling for nursing to double their PhD graduates by 2020, but not all PhD programs in nursing have content specific to nursing education. Therefore, being a PhD-prepared nurse does not automatically provide you with the needed skills of scholarship presentation.

Graduate nurse educator tracks are more apt to focus on the academic environment but many times only touch the surface of what will be expected of nurse educators from the larger educational organization. The National League for Nursing's Core Competencies for Nurse Educators (NLN, 2005) dedicates Competency 8—Function within the Educational Environment—to skills specific to nurse educators' roles in educational organization. This emphasizes the importance of the nurse educators' ability to be scholarly, contributing members of the larger educational organization.

## SUMMARY

A well-thought-out academic portfolio is needed when you, the nurse educator, present yourself for an academic position, promotion, or tenure because you are being critiqued by academic standards as opposed to familiar health care standards. There are also personal and professional reasons that academic portfolios are becoming increasingly important:

- The clear articulation of your philosophy of education
- Educating academics from other disciplines about the scholarship of nursing

Nurses will be moving increasingly into collegiate positions due to a combination of social forces that include:

- The current IOM report to increase the BSN workforce
- ANCC's Magnet Recognition Program®
- BSN in 10 Movement
- Research discussion educational preparation related to patient mortality and morbidity (Aiken et al., 2003)

Once in collegiate settings, nurse educators should be aware of the differences inherent in their profession when considering the presentation of their academic portfolio. Some of those differences include nursing's:

- Relatively short academic history
- Diverse teaching environments including classroom, clinical, and laboratory
- Lack of consistency about entry into practice
- History of being a female-dominated profession
- Trend of educators entering academia later than educators from other disciplines
- Program outcome evaluation process, which uses the success percentages of NCLEX-RN®

The combination of all of these factors makes an effective academic portfolio a must in order for you to secure an academic position or apply for promotion or tenure.

# 2

## Background

### What Is the Story and Purpose Behind Your Academic Portfolio?

## INTRODUCTION

*Portfolios can demonstrate professional and personal growth for nurse educators. Much has been much written about using portfolios to demonstrate the achievement of learning outcomes for students (Lewallen & Kohlenberg, 2011), but less has been written and studied about the use of academic portfolios for nurse educators. Some of the principles are the same, even if the evidence for and the purpose of the portfolios differ. This chapter will briefly discuss the history of academic portfolios and highlight the few studies that have been conducted about them.*

At the end of this chapter, the nurse educator will be able to:

1. Explain the historical development of academic portfolios.
2. Appraise the current evidence related to academic portfolios.
3. Discuss the three main purposes of developing an academic portfolio.

21

## THE HISTORY OF PORTFOLIOS

The idea of portfolios was borrowed from artists and architects. It was not until the 1980s that the idea was proposed as a method to demonstrate individual faculty accomplishments (Melland & Volden, 1996). Due to the complex role of an academic educator, portfolios are an excellent method to demonstrate the multifaceted scholarship of educators.

Originally academic portfolios were called "teaching portfolios" and indeed that phrase is still appropriate if a nurse educator is concentrating just on educational excellence. More often in academia today scholarship also needs to be displayed in the areas of research and service. The teaching portfolio "serves to document a faculty member's commitment to and accomplishments relative to the scholarship of teaching" (Reece, Pearce, Melillo, & Beaudry, 2001, p. 182).

Seldin and Miller (2009) use anecdotal evidence to support the fact that academic portfolios improve performance and assist in personal career decisions. Through personal testimonies they demonstrate that portfolios have assisted people for promotion, tenure, and post-tenure review. More subjectively their testimonies from portfolio developers show personal growth through terms that describe them as "eye-opening," "tying threads together," a chance to "refocus," and "stepping back" to gain the larger perspective of one's own career path (p. 7). All professionals feel that, at some point in their careers, they are running on a treadmill and need to stop and stand on firm ground in order to take in that panoramic view of their personal and professional goals.

═══════════════════════*FAST FACTS* in a *NUTSHELL*

The physical and cognitive exercise of gathering, categorizing, labeling, and explaining evidence that is specific to the individual is a retreat into the past that allows you to identify strengths and deficiencies, reflect on them, and then set goals for the future.

## EVIDENCE OF PORTFOLIO OUTCOMES

Although there is more research concerning student portfolios than academic portfolios, some of the student-focused studies have provided us with valuable information. Portfolios have been described as valuable tools to assist students to meet their learning goals, as well as to promote critical thinking (O'Mara, Carpio, Mallette, Down, & Brown, 2000).

McColgan and Blackwood (2009) did a systematic review of the use of teaching portfolios and found a wide variety, sometimes under terms such as "academic dossier" and "interfolio" (p. 2505). The review of the search protocol did identify that although portfolios are now more widely used, there is mostly anecdotal evidence related to their outcomes. Future study recommendations will inevitably focus on outcome research.

Other practice-grounded disciplines have studied the extent of portfolio usage in academia. Luk, Yukawa, and Emery (2009) surveyed *clinician-educators* ($n = 125$) and department chairs ($n = 10$) on the use of portfolios. The results from this study demonstrated that only two department chairs stated they provided education for faculty to assist them in portfolio preparation and that 86% of faculty respondents did not receive any information on how to develop their portfolio. Also interesting was the finding that 48% did not know the difference between a portfolio and other types of faculty evaluation tools. This supports the findings of McColgan and Blackwood (2009), which stated that academic portfolios are a relatively new evaluation mechanism.

Driessen, Van Tartwijk, and Van Der Vleuten (2007) wrote a systematic review of the use of portfolios as an evaluative tool for medical education. Although this study focused on student portfolios, the conclusions drawn from multiple studies were noteworthy for all portfolio development:

- Further studies on effectiveness are warranted.
- Portfolios have characteristics of holistic assessment.
- The competencies of the portfolio mentor are important.

O'Mara, Carpio, Mallette, Down, and Brown (2000) completed a pilot study ($n = 10$) using content analysis as a qualitative method to capture key ideas. Three major themes occurred: taking stock, documenting practice, and reflection. Taking stock was a theme that required nurse educators to take a risk and make their teaching accomplishments and needs for improvement visible. Documenting practice was seen as a process for writing all that was involved in collegiate teaching and curriculum development and for revealing the vast extent of the participant's involvement. Reflection occurred throughout the process and generated feelings of discomfort at times because of the exposure that reflective writing produces. The conclusion to the study not only explained the individual benefits to the participants, but the peer and team benefits of developing academic portfolios together.

As you can see from the few studies that have been done on academic portfolios, more information on their development and outcomes is needed. Academic portfolios have also served more than one purpose for the participants of the studies, and those purposes will be expanded upon in the next section of this chapter.

## PORTFOLIO PURPOSE #1: PERSONAL GROWTH

Nursing education is changing as quickly as the practice setting and is demanding new tasks of all educators. This is reflected in the statement of Alteen, Didham, and Stratton (2009).

The literature as well as current trends supports the fact that there has never been a stronger case for nurse educators to revisit their own values, beliefs, and assumptions about teaching and scholarship to more effectively embrace the challenges of academia (p. 268).

All nurse educators progress through the stages from novice to expert (Benner, 1984). This is easy to observe in teachers who, with experience, progress from simply reading from notes and PowerPoint® slides to focused classroom discussions and dissection of case studies.

═══════════════*FAST FACTS in a NUTSHELL*

Portfolios are a face-to-face reflection and evaluation of an educator's work.

Portfolio evidence presents growth by examples or explanation. It can also serve as a:

...springboard for performance improvement. It is in the very process of reflecting on their own work and creating the collection of documents and materials that the professor is stimulated to reconsider policies and activities, rethink strategies and methodologies, revise priorities, and plan for the future. (Seldin & Miller, 2009, p. 4)

Therefore, the suggestion of starting a portfolio early, even when it is not needed for employment or promotion, is a great idea. It can serve as an ongoing process for self-reflection and be developed as a direct reflection of your personal career development. Additionally, it will make it easier when needed for employment or promotion.

## PORTFOLIO PURPOSE #2: PROFESSIONAL GROWTH

Academic portfolios are a mechanism for novice and expert nurse educators to demonstrate professional growth. "It brings together information about a professor's most significant professional accomplishments" (Seldin & Miller, 2009, p. 2). It is the tool you need to sell yourself. Therefore, it is very important to choose the evidence to include carefully, depending upon the nurse educator's stage of career or the purpose of the portfolio. For example, Lewallen and Kohlenberg (2011) discuss preparing doctoral students for the role of academics by preparing a "career portfolio" (p. 24). The career portfolio for doctoral students aspiring to teach in academia includes key elements to showcase their accomplishments:

- Curriculum vitae
- Teaching philosophy
- Career plan
- Identified possible funding sources (grants)
- PowerPoint® presentation(s) that they have used for a teaching session

Professional growth demonstration will be different for each individual depending upon:

- Purpose of the portfolio
- Career stage
- Mission of the institution for which it is being reviewed, which will be discussed in depth in Chapter 3

As stated, each portfolio is very individualized, but the reviewer of the portfolio should be able to glean immediately the purpose and intent of the portfolio. There should be a clear match between the purpose of the portfolio and the contents of the portfolio.

## PORTFOLIO PURPOSE #3: A TEACHING TOOL FOR NON-NURSE ACADEMICS

A third important purpose of a nurse educator's portfolio is to increase the understanding of the scholarship of nursing for other academic scholars. Hopefully nurse educators are part of the evaluative committee in case explanations are warranted. Nursing is a young and different discipline in academia. We are preparing professionals that are skilled as knowledge workers who directly care for humans in high-risk situations. This mission sets us apart from other disciplines; thus, nurse educators obviously need to use methodologies that are not used by other disciplines. This is especially true when considering the scholarship of clinical teaching, which includes on-site clinical teaching, case studies, and simulation.

Also, other academic educators may not be aware of the classifications of nursing journals, publications, conferences, and standards of accrediting and regulating organizations. Most other disciplines do not teach undergraduate learners who can be pre-licensure and post-licensure, as well as working toward a second degree. All of these issues, which are second nature to nurse educators, may be foreign to educators in other disciplines and the carefully crafted portfolio can be a mechanism to educate as well as evaluate.

## PERSONAL EXPERIENCE: ANECDOTAL EVIDENCE

The author's current administrative position allowed her the privilege of assisting four nurse educators in the development of their academic portfolios. Two portfolios were developed for promotion from Instructor to Assistant Professor and two were developed to secure tenure. All four promotions were granted. Parts of those current, successful portfolios will be shared as examples throughout this book.

## SUMMARY

As can be gleaned, more research, both quantitative and qualitative, is needed on the development, process, and outcome evaluation of academic portfolios both for students and faculty. Anecdotally academic portfolio development is supported as an effective reflective and evaluative mechanism for nurse educators. Portfolios are developed to serve three distinct yet interwoven purposes. To this end, there has not been a better evaluative tool developed to showcase the scholarship of nurse educators. Therefore the next chapter will discuss how to use your portfolio to assess your academic environment as well as your career development and goals.

# 3

## Assessment

### Assessing the Academic Environment and Your Career Goals

## INTRODUCTION

*Developing a career trajectory in academia is essential in order to guide the development of your specific areas of scholarship. It is as equally important to understand the academic environment for which you are interviewing or hope to advance. Your career development plan should fit your current institution so that expectations and accomplishments are cohesive. This will lead to a well-integrated career plan and increase the probability of your success.*

## FAST FACTS in a NUTSHELL

"Successful faculty members have often developed a career developmental plan for themselves."
(Glasgow, 2009, p. 221)

At the end of this chapter, the nurse educator will be able to:

1. Reflect on personal career goals.
2. Differentiate between missions of different institutions.
3. Assess the match between goals and mission.

## DEVELOPING A CAREER TRAJECTORY

To develop a realistic career trajectory, it is helpful to write down attainable short- and long-term career goals. Not only should these goals be well thought out and realistic but they should be revisited often. As a rule of thumb, short-term goals are those things that you wish to accomplish within a couple of months to 1 year. Goals such as submit an abstract for presentation or add an active teaching strategy next semester are good short-term goals. Long-term goals can usually be accomplished within 2 to 6 years. A long-term goal may be to finish your terminal degree in nursing or advance from an instructor to an assistant professor.

*FAST FACTS in a NUTSHELL*

Along with writing down both short- and long-term goals, you will need to make a calendar to ensure effective time management.

Some tips on time management include:

• Identify the time of day when you get the most work accomplished and protect it.
• Place a high value on the piece of scholarship (teaching, research/publications, service) you need most

to promote your success, and attend to that piece first.
- Say "No" if others want to get you involved in their goals and that do not foster your goals.
- It is okay to say "No" and protect your time because in the end only you are accountable for your own career goals.

═══════════════════════════*FAST FACTS in a NUTSHELL*

It is easier to decline assisting someone else if you develop an honest, pre-contemplated response such as. "I would love to help you but right now my plate is full. I am working on several projects that I need to complete. If you'd like we can discuss this again in a few months."

Other important points in your self-assessment process have been articulated by Glasgow (2009):

- Master negotiating skills as well as conflict-resolution skills.
- Develop collaboration skills and the ability to maximize the benefits of collaboration while maintaining autonomy and boundaries.
- Develop a primary mentor–protégé relationship. (p. 222)

## BEING MENTORED

Many institutions assign a mentor to promote academic success. Other times, nurse educators must seek out their own mentors. Mentors can be from the same department but do not have to be. There are advantages and disadvantages to both models. In either case it should be formalized as a collaborative relationship that includes consultation and coaching. A mentoring relationship is more than just helping a colleague with a project—it is an ongoing, reciprocal relationship.

*FAST FACTS in a NUTSHELL*

Grossman and Valiga (2005) include as a mentor's job assisting the protégé in establishing a professional reputation in the organization.

Your mentor can also assist you in understanding the political environment of the institution in which you are interviewing for employment or petitioning for promotion (Glasgow, 2009).

Mentors can be instrumental in assisting you in developing your academic portfolio. With a mentor's guidance you can collect evidence, reflect upon it, and choose the most significant evidence for integration into the end product.

## THE EXPECTATIONS OF THE INSTITUTION

Know the expectations of the institution. Different types of universities and colleges have different academic emphasis depending upon their mission. The Carnegie Foundation for the Advancement of Teaching (2010) maintains a basic classification of different types of colleges (Exhibit 3.1).

**Exhibit 3.1**    The Carnegie Foundation for the Advancement of Teaching: Basic Classifications of Schools of Higher Education in the United States

- Assoc/Pub-R-S: Associate's–Public Rural-serving Small
- Assoc/Pub-R-M: Associate's–Public Rural-serving Medium
- Assoc/Pub-R-L: Associate's–Public Rural-serving Large
- Assoc/Pub-S-SC: Associate's–Public Suburban-serving Single Campus
- Assoc/Pub-S-MC: Associate's–Public Suburban-serving Multicampus
- Assoc/Pub-U-SC: Associate's–Public Urban-serving Single Campus
- Assoc/Pub-U-MC: Associate's–Public Urban-serving Multicampus
- Assoc/Pub-Spec: Associate's–Public Special Use
- Assoc/PrivNFP: Associate's–Private Not-for-profit
- Assoc/PrivFP: Associate's–Private For-profit
- Assoc/Pub2in4: Associate's–Public 2-year colleges under 4-year universities
- Assoc/Pub4: Associate's–Public 4-year Primarily Associate's
- Assoc/PrivNFP4: Associate's–Private Not-for-profit 4-year Primarily Associate's

*Continued*

**Exhibit 3.1**  *Continued*

- Assoc/PrivFP4: Associate's–Private For-profit 4-year Primarily Associate's
- RU/VH: Research Universities (very high research activity)
- RU/H: Research Universities (high research activity)
- DRU: Doctoral/Research Universities
- Master's L: Master's Colleges and Universities (larger programs)
- Master's M: Master's Colleges and Universities (medium programs)
- Master's S: Master's Colleges and Universities (smaller programs)
- Bac/A&S: Baccalaureate Colleges–Arts & Sciences
- Bac/Diverse: Baccalaureate Colleges–Diverse Fields
- Bac/Assoc: Baccalaureate/Associate's Colleges
- Spec/Faith: Special Focus Institutions–Theological seminaries, Bible colleges, and other faith-related institutions
- Spec/Med: Special Focus Institutions–Medical schools and medical centers
- Spec/Health: Special Focus Institutions–Other health professions schools
- Spec/Engg: Special Focus Institutions–Schools of engineering
- Spec/Tech: Special Focus Institutions–Other technology-related schools
- Spec/Bus: Special Focus Institutions–Schools of business and management

*Continued*

**Exhibit 3.1**  *Continued*

- Spec/Arts: Special Focus Institutions–Schools of art, music, and design
- Spec/Law: Special Focus Institutions–Schools of law
- Spec/Other: Special Focus Institutions–Other special-focus institutions
- Tribal: Tribal Colleges

*Source:* Reprinted with permission of the Carnegie Foundation for the Advancement of Teaching; retrieved from http://classifications.carnegiefoundation.org/lookup_listings

═══════════════*FAST FACTS in a NUTSHELL*

It is important to know the classification of your institution for academic portfolio development.

For example, if your nursing program is part of a baccalaureate college of arts and sciences (Bac/A&S), the focus will be on the scholarship areas of teaching and service and this should be described most fully in your portfolio. If the nursing program in which you teach is in a university with high research activity (RU/H), then your academic portfolio will have more concentrated information on the scholarship of research. It is important for you to know the expectations of your governing organization or the one to which you are applying prior to embarking on the development of an academic portfolio.

## THE INSTITUTION'S MISSION

The institution's mission will be connected to its Carnegie classification. Therefore, if it is classified as a Bac/A&S: Baccalaureate Colleges–Arts & Sciences, you would expect the mission statement of the institution to reflect the fact that it bases its curriculum on a firm foundation of liberal arts and sciences. If it is a public college (state administrated and financed), it may have as part of its mission to serve the area. Another example is institutions that are in the research category. The mission statement would reflect its intent to develop and disseminate original knowledge. The mission statement of the College/School/Department of Nursing will stem from the mission of the institution. Large colleges of nursing may be research driven while other schools may focus on teaching the next generation of professional nurses.

- Do you know what the University/College and the College/School/Department of Nursing mission statements are?

## THE MISSION OF THE DEPARTMENT OF NURSING

The Department/School/College of Nursing within the institution is also driven by a mission statement. The mission for nursing is usually more specific but is never in conflict with the institutional mission. An example is "to use the strong foundations of a liberal arts education in order to educate baccalaureate prepared nurses to service the local area." Your short- and long-term goals should also be synchronous with the mission of your department.

**═══════════════════════════════════════FAST FACTS in a NUTSHELL**

Know your institution's classification and mission, as well as your department's mission statement.

## ACADEMIC TRACKS

As mentioned in Chapter 1, two very important resources are the institution's faculty handbook and the department of nursing's faculty handbook. These provide the information you need to understand the hiring, promotion, and tenure policies of the institution. They should be followed as closely as possible when you make a career move. The policies will specify what documents they expect you to present for a career move and when they expect them.

**═══════════════════════════════════════FAST FACTS in a NUTSHELL**

- Most colleges and universities have firm deadlines for applications regarding hiring and promotion.
- The faculty and department handbooks for your academic setting should become your best friends when preparing for a career move.

The categories of academic positions may differ from institution to institution, but the main categories and the general expected skill sets are listed in Table 3.1.

## TABLE 3.1　Common Academic Positions and Accompanying Skill Sets

| Title | Skill Set |
| --- | --- |
| Instructor | Develop skills in the scholarship of teaching.<br>Begin to develop skills in research.<br>Provide service to the educational unit.<br>Understand the responsibilities of protégé and mentor. |
| Assistant Professor | Develop an area of expertise.<br>Pose and address an important question or focus in that area that has the potential for significant findings or impact (scholarship or research).<br>Promote service to the educational unit and the institution.<br>Lead or collaborate in the development and evaluation of an educational program.<br>Present findings from this work at appropriate national meetings and/or publish the results of this work in peer-reviewed journals.<br>Obtain internal or external, peer-reviewed funding to support this work. |
| Associate Professor | Continue research/scholarship in one's area of expertise as an autonomous investigator and in publication productivity.<br>Become an interdependent investigator and/or leader.<br>Continue in the development and evaluation of educational programs.<br>Become nationally and internationally recognized for this work. Take on responsibility in an important role for one's own institution.<br>Mentor junior faculty in a productive manner.<br>Serve on national committees.<br>Serve on departmental and university functions, particularly some time-consuming committees. |
| Professor | Continue leadership in research, teaching, and service.<br>Function as a role model.<br>Enhance your mentoring role and, in particular, assist junior faculty in their career development. |

*Source:* Adapted from Glasgow, M. E. S. (2009). Functioning effectively within the institutional environment and academic community. In R. A. Wittmann-Price & M. Godshall (Eds.), *Certified nurse educator (CNE) review manual* (pp. 213–231). New York: Springer Publishing Company. Reprinted with permission.

## ASSESSING THE MATCH

Your short- and long-term career goals should be synchronous with the institution's and department's missions. For
example, if you are a researcher and would like to spend
at least 50% of your academic time on clinical research,
then you will probably be frustrated in an institution that

Name _____

| Short-Term Career Goals | | Date of Accomplishment | | |
|---|---|---|---|---|
| 1. | | | | |
| 2. | | | | |
| 3. | | | | |
| Long-Term Career Goals | | | | |
| | | | | |
| Institution's Classification | | | | |
| | | | | |
| Institution's Main Mission | | | | |
| | | | | |
| Department's Main Mission | | | | |
| | | | | |
| Assess the Match Between Your Goals and the Institution's Mission | | | | |
| 5 | 4 | 3 | 2 | 1 |
| Perfect match; this is where I was meant to be. | Good match; I can make this job work for me. | Not such a good match, but I might make it work. | Poor match; it will be a struggle to make it work. | Does not match at all and I will be setting myself up for failure. |
| Do I need to adjust my short- or long-term goals? Why? | | | | |

is primarily a baccalaureate college of arts and science with the primary function of education. If your passion is teaching, then you may not fit well in a research intensive institution. An honest assessment of your goals and the institution's goals is invaluable to promote your career success. Use the checklist on page 39 to begin your assessment of how well your goals and the goals of your institution "match."

## SUMMARY

Before embarking on academic portfolio development, it is imperative that you place mindful thought into specific areas of career assessment:

- What are my professional and personal goals?
- What are the expectations of the institution?
- Do the expectations and the goals match or will they match in the near future?

During this assessment phase of your career, it may help to talk over your thoughts and intentions with other nurse educators and your mentor who may have been in the academic realm for a longer period of time. They may be able to impart the practical wisdom needed to supplement the procedural knowledge found in the faculty handbooks. Chapter 4 will discuss what evidence to start collecting and how.

# 4

# Recommendations

## Laying the Foundation to Begin the Process

## INTRODUCTION

*Now that the purpose and significance of an academic portfolio have been fully explored, the next step is a recommended plan of action. The plan of action is simple—just get started collecting the evidence and writing the sections. Once the personal statements are written, they are much easier to update and manipulate than starting from scratch when it is time to submit it for promotion or tenure. So this chapter will provide you with recommendations to get you started.*

At the end of this chapter, the nurse educator will be able to:

1. Develop a time schedule for academic portfolio updating.
2. Demonstrate organization of evidence.
3. Provide a rationale for collecting specific pieces of evidence.

## SETTING A SCHEDULE

Imperative to accomplishing any large academic task is setting a schedule and holding yourself accountable to it. Know your best time of day for critical thinking. Many individuals are more cognitively alert in the morning, while others function best in the evening. The schedule should contain uninterrupted time to organize your thoughts and put career goals into perspective.

### FAST FACTS in a NUTSHELL

Schedule time for developing your academic portfolio and record it in the calendar that you use all the time.

"How often?" is always another question asked when an ongoing task needs to be accomplished. You know best how you yourself "chunk" time. If you are a person that likes smaller portions of time, then schedule it once a week. Others are fine collecting information and writing once a month.

### FAST FACTS in a NUTSHELL

Start to view time as expandable rather than limiting—just fit it in and it will fit. If you worry about how to fit it in, it will not happen.

## ORGANIZE YOUR EFFORTS

Once you have scheduled the time to work on your portfolio, you then need two types of secured space. You need space for your electronic work and space for your hard copies of evidence unless you are going to scan all documents. Personal computers that are not organized and loaded with files making it easy to lose important documents. A small flash drive, specifically for your academic portfolio, is a good idea for several reasons. If you change your academic employment position, the flash drive is easy to take along. If your personal computer is disrupted, your portfolio will be safe. But of course, like all documents, it should be backed up.

The second space is physical space to collect items that you may decide to use as evidence. A locked drawer, specific for this purpose, works well. The lock is not needed as much for safety as it is to secure the documents from being stored and lost among other documents. The physical activity required to lock and unlock the drawer encourages you to think about the importance of the evidence that you are collecting.

## PROCURE AN ACADEMIC BUDDY

Having another nurse educator working on his or her portfolio during the same time period is invaluable. You can set up times to discuss what is important, how things should be phrased, and to provide constructive critique of each other's work along the way. Many people are more productive when working with another or others. Creating small groups within a department who work together collegially, but separately, on their portfolios can be a productive strategy for all involved.

═══════════════════════*FAST FACTS in a NUTSHELL*

Going up for promotion and tenure is a stressful life situation. Working as a group can decrease the stress.

## START COLLECTING

Collect the things that you think may show your scholarship. Even if you do not ultimately use them all, when you can compare your evidence to what you have written you can make the best choices. If you do something that might be applicable to your finished product, such as "I interviewed five honor students for scholarships today," be sure to write it down with the date in case you eventually incorporate it into your academic portfolio.

*FAST FACTS in a NUTSHELL*

If the items or documents you collect need to be used for yearly evaluations, don't forget to make high quality copies.

## SUMMARY

Now that the situation, background, and assessment of an academic portfolio are clear, the recommendations are simple and to the point. First, make a schedule to work on your academic portfolio. Second, secure space and, if possible, engage a buddy or small group to embark on the task with you. Finally, start collecting evidence! The next part of the book goes into detail about how to develop your academic portfolio, discussing the personal statement, which is the main portion of your academic portfolio, and breaking it down into manageable parts. It gives hints on actually putting the physical academic portfolio together. In order to clarify the task at hand, examples are provided along the way.

# The How of Developing Your
# Academic Portfolio

# 5

## How to Write a Five-Part Personal Statement

### INTRODUCTION

*Your personal statement is the main part of the portfolio. Some institutions limit the number of pages for this paramount piece but most do not. The personal statement must be accurate, concise, clear, and a highlight of accomplishments, and not an exhaustive manuscript of everything that you have ever done. Because every educator and institution of employment is different, no two academic portfolios will look the same, but there are some important common pieces. This chapter will begin to discuss those important pieces starting with the personal statement.*

At the end of this chapter, the nurse educator will be able to:

1. Understand the importance of the personal statement.
2. List the parts of a personal statement.
3. Decide if the description of your teaching, research, or service should follow the preface in your personal statement.

## THE PERSONAL STATEMENT

The personal statement is an essay and is the first piece of information your evaluator will read when they open your portfolio. Unless the portfolio is for a first job, the personal statement should reflect the accomplishments that have occurred while the nurse educator has been in the current position. The personal statement is divided into five parts and the discussion of each part will be expanded in order to underscore the significance of each. The five parts are:

- Part 1: Preface/Abstract
- Part 2: Teaching
- Part 3: Research and/or Scholarship
- Part 4: Service
- Part 5: Integrative Summary

========================= *FAST FACTS in a NUTSHELL*

The length of your personal statement may be dictated by your institution. Some institutions even have different length requirements for promotion versus tenure. This information will be in your faculty handbook. The average length of a personal statement can range from 10 to 20 pages.

## PART I: THE PREFACE/ABSTRACT

It is important to state the specific purpose of the portfolio right in the beginning of the portfolio. This provides clear intent to the reviewer or reader. Some of the reasons to develop the portfolio may be:

- First academic job or practice
- Promotion

- Midpoint review (usually the third year of employment) between hire and application for tenure
- Tenure

The preface does not have to be more than a half a page, but up to a full page is acceptable. In the event that the portfolio is being used for a first job, the preface is often in the form of a cover letter.

═══════════════════════════════════*FAST FACTS in a NUTSHELL*

The preface or abstract part of your personal statement tells the evaluator(s) exactly why you are submitting your portfolio.

For promotion and tenure portfolios, the scholarship areas of teaching, research, and service are mentioned in the preface in order for the reviewer/reader to know what to expect. The actual expansion and elaboration will be done in the sections following the preface. Exhibit 5.1 is the preface taken from the author's midpoint review (i.e., the 3-year mark in a 6-year tenure track position); it is one single-spaced page that sets the stage for the rest of the author's personal statement:

**Exhibit 5.1**   Preface to My Personal Statement

The purpose of this portfolio is to highlight my academic accomplishments for my mid-point review. Now that I have been a faculty member for over 2 years, I am very encouraged by the professional

*Continued*

**Exhibit 5.1**  *Continued*

atmosphere and the support I have received to reach my mid-point evaluation.

My research activities (50% effort) include a $1000.00 grant from the Honor Society. I am also working on a grant with the Rheumatology Department to fund a bone health nurse at (the associated hospital) and an internal grant with the Sports Management faculty. My scholarship has flourished since I began my career at this university. I have published two books in 2 years (*Certified Nurse Educator (CNE) Review Manual* and *NCLEX-RN® EXCEL: Test Success Through Unfolding Case Study Review,* 2009 and 2010, Springer Publishing Company). I have published five peer-reviewed articles and two chapters. I have presented nationally and locally, and was invited to present internationally.

I have had numerous teaching opportunities to develop multiple aspects of my faculty position. In the realm of teaching (30% effort), I was awarded the **Nursing Spectrum's Regional Award for Excellence in Education** in May of 2008. I have successfully taught undergraduate Women's Health and I am a guest lecturer for all the NICU lectures regardless of who is the primary instructor. I am also the guest lecturer for many senior review courses for women's health, and have developed unfolding case studies using clicker technology in order to create an active learning atmosphere. I have also taught at the graduate level (Nurse Educator) and I am currently teaching DrNP students. I have been awarded **Coordinator of the Education Track** because of my expertise as a Certified Nurse Educator (CNE). I am

*Continued*

**Exhibit 5.1**  *Continued*

also the course chair on the Contemporary Nurse Educator Practicum. I recently (June 2009) published a review manual for the CNE examination. I am dissertation chair for a doctoral student and qualifying exam advisor for another doctoral student.

As part of my teaching expectations (20% effort), I teach evidence-based practice (EBP) to staff nurses. I oversee nine IRB-approved projects. I have assisted nursing administrators to develop and submit the necessary documents for Magnet® status to the AACN (American Association of Colleges of Nursing) and have developed an ongoing Evidence-Based Leadership Program that will enroll six more staff nurses in October of 2009.

My service to the university and hospital has been multifaceted. My university service includes serving on the student conduct committee (1 year), the curriculum committee (2 years), grade distribution ad-hoc committee, informatics position interview committee, publication club contributor, and I was just elected to Faculty Advisory Council. I meet and exceed my faculty requirements for proctoring and recruiting. I provide administrative coverage to the doctoral program when the chair is unavailable. My service to the hospital system includes serving on the Nurse Executive Council, Steering Committee, and presenting at in-services and symposiums. My service also extends to the community. I work at the local free clinic every Wednesday; I assess patients, educate families, and refer health care issues.

*Continued*

**Exhibit 5.1**    *Continued*

My midpoint review of my first 2 years of employment has provided me with the opportunity to reflect on the vast amount of personal growth I have acquired.

*FAST FACTS in a NUTSHELL*

Set the stage for the evaluator(s)—do not let them guess why you are submitting.

Now the evaluator(s) are aware that this is a 2-year compilation of material for a mid-point evaluation. It was developed with the assistance of my mentor.

*FAST FACTS in a NUTSHELL*

It takes approximately four to five revisions of the personal statement between you and your mentor to refine it so that it showcases your accomplishments in the best light!

The preface to this personal statement also tells the evaluator(s) how the rest of the personal statement and then the portfolio will be arranged. It communicates that 50% effort is devoted to research and the other 50% effort is devoted to teaching, split (30/20) between two institutions. Because this preface was developed for a research intensive (DR-INT) institution, the research portion of the personal statement and the portfolio should come first. It also coordinates with the university's mission statement. The university also has a research mission statement which makes it clear that for an academic position to be successful within the university, research should be highlighted. If you are compiling an academic portfolio for the purpose of being hired primarily as a teacher, the teaching section would precede the research, scholarship, or service sections of the personal statement and at the portfolio sections. The same would be true for the service section if the nurse educator has a position such as coordinator for service learning,

The following (Exhibit 5.2) is a preface used for the purpose of seeking a first academic job. It is in the form of a cover letter to introduce the portfolio but it is very effective in telling the interview team exactly the purpose of the application.

**Exhibit 5.2**   First Job Personal Statement

Greetings!
I am writing you to apply for the Nursing Instructor Position at your university. I am interested in this position because I have heard wonderful reviews from both students and faculty at your educational institution. I have a passion for nursing education and have been a preceptor many time on the labor and delivery unit in which I work. I am enrolled in MSN in Nursing Education and am anxious to put the theory I have learned about teaching and learning into practice. The prospect of facilitating learning in the next generation of nurses is a lifelong dream. I have a strong and attentive work ethic, participate well with others, and have a very positive attitude. I feel that I could be an asset to your educational mission, as I promise to work hard as a nurse

*Continued*

**Exhibit 5.2**  *Continued*

educator in this ever-changing multicultural world that longs to receive extraordinary health care from the nurses I will teach. Thank you for your time, and I look forward to hearing from you!

With best regards,
Jeana Dunn

This personal statement, in the form of a cover letter, was the first piece of information in the portfolio and informs the interview team that the apaplicant is a novice educator who has an MSN and is pursuing an entry-level instructor role. It also gives the interview team an idea of enthusiasm which is important for both position requests and promotion.

Exhibit 5.3 is a preface from Dr. Rhonda Brogdon's personal statement which was successfully used for promotion.

**Exhibit 5.3**  Personal Statement for Promotion

I, Rhonda Brogdon, am applying for Assistant Professor/tenure-track and will outline my 5-year record of excellence in teaching, scholarship, and service to Francis Marion University. I worked for the MUSC-FMU satellite nursing program from 2002–2004 as a part-time clinical instructor. I have chosen to continue my career here because I am impressed with the support FMU provides to its faculty and the University's dedication to providing outstanding education to students that supports the mission and

*Continued*

**Exhibit 5.3** *Continued*

vision of the institution. In the past 5 years, I have fulfilled the criteria for Assistant Professor by demonstrating excellence in teaching, professional scholarship, and service to both my profession as well as the University while completing my Doctorate in Nursing Practice. In 2007, I was awarded the Caring Clinical Instructor Award from the 2007 May nursing graduates and in 2008; I was inducted into Francis Marion's University Department of Nursing Honor Society. The following sections of my personal statement will provide detailed description regarding my excellence in teaching which spans multiple courses for the department of nursing, my scholarship which includes the completion of a clinical project for my terminal degree, and my service to the department, university, and community.

Once you have the preface to your personal statement completed you are ready to move on to the next section (Part 2) of your personal statement. For most academic portfolios the next section will be about your scholarship in teaching, but this may depend on the type of institution to which you are applying or requesting promotion. Chapter 6 will describe in depth the teaching part of the personal statement and the evidence that you will need to support the claims you make.

## SUMMARY

This chapter introduced you to the most important part of your academic portfolio, your personal statement. The chapter provided an explanation of the first part of the personal statement, the preface or abstract, which sets the stage for the rest of the portfolio contents and tells the reviewers exactly why you are submitting your academic portfolio.

=== FAST FACTS in a NUTSHELL

Ongoing outline of your academic portfolio:

1.  Part I: Preface/Abstract (approximately 1 page)

# 6

# How to Showcase Your Teaching

## INTRODUCTION

*It is likely that the next section or Part 2 of your personal statement will be about your teaching scholarship and will explain to the interview team or the reviewers why you are an excellent teacher who facilitates learning and inquiry. This should be done with accuracy, conciseness, and confidence. Examples of "teaching" sections of educators' personal statements are provided.*

At the end of this chapter, the nurse educator will be able to:

1. Discuss important components to include in the teaching section of your personal statement.
2. Develop a teaching philosophy.
3. Select evidence that will support the claims made in your personal statement.

## OVERVIEW OF THE TEACHING SECTION

As stated, the length of the personal section may be man-
dated by your university, but usually it is approximately
five pages in length. Teaching sections may be a bit shorter,
averaging two to three pages.

## TEACHING PHILOSOPHY

Your teaching philosophy is the first section of *Part 2:
Teaching* of your personal statement.

*FAST FACTS in a NUTSHELL*

Your teaching philosophy should be congruent with
the missions of the institution and the educational
unit.

According to Alteen, Didham, and Stratton (2009), who
reference Sweitzer (2003), your teaching philosophy
should include the following components:

- Your knowledge and values about teaching and
  learning.
- How learning takes place for the learner and why.
- What learners bring to the teaching/learning
  environment.
- What teachers bring to the teaching/learning
  environment.

═══════════════════════════*FAST FACTS in a NUTSHELL*

"Teaching philosophy is a statement of beliefs about teaching and learning, learners, classroom and clinical teaching strategies, the educator's role, and how scholarly work and service integrate with the teaching focus." (Billings & Kowalski, 2008, p. 533)

Specifically, your philosophy should not be more than one page of *Part 2: Teaching* of your personal statement. As an example, my teaching philosophy is provided in Exhibit 6.1.

**Exhibit 6.1**   Teaching Philosophy

My teaching is based on the theory developed by Paulo Freire (1970) who proposed that educational institutions are powerful enough to promote an emancipated society. He expanded on the description of social norms that oppress and included the educational environment. Freire believed that oppression serves the purpose of dehumanization by producing a "culture of silence" that is exploited for political or economic gain. Because of this intellectual, emotional, and psychological enslavement, the oppressed develop a "fear of freedom" (Freire, 1970, p. 36) in exchange for perceived security.

The outcome of emancipated education for any group is to equalize power between information

*Continued*

**Exhibit 6.1**    *Continued*

giver and receiver in order to enable free choice and create an environment of true humanism that may extend into all social systems (Freire, 1970, 1992, 1998). It was not until I read Freire's (1970) *Pedagogy of the Oppressed* that I seriously considered the social aspect as a determinate of the educational stance of people. The methodologies proposed by Freire as necessary infusions into the classroom create an equalitarian society of learning for both the educator and the learner. Freire proposes the establishment of a collaborative climate in which students take responsibility for their learning.

One of the main components of Freire's Emancipatory Education model is reflection and is characterized by critically thinking about alternatives. Reflection can take the form of interpersonal dialogue or self-dialogue, both producing an internal awareness. Freire believed that traditional educational methods alone foster oppression because they do not encourage the reflection needed for critical thinking (Romyn, 2000). It is important to reflect on issues in order to recognize the inherent personal and social aspects. Reflection is also needed to critically think about the information gained from personal and empirical knowledge in order to synthesize it into a decision (Fahrenfort, 1987).

From the teaching philosophy presented in Exhibit 6.1, you would expect to see several threads carried through the teaching section of the academic portfolio. Reflection has been identified as important; therefore, evidence might be included of a student's reflection that demonstrates critical thinking. A syllabus might also be included in the appendix to the portfolio that weighs discussion as an important component in evaluation methods used to demonstrate teaching philosophy in action.

========================*FAST FACTS in a NUTSHELL*

The appendices in your portfolio are the best examples of evidence that will support your personal statement.

First-time academics may have a philosophy that is more directed toward clinical care, especially if they are going to enter academia as clinical instructors initially. Exhibit 6.2 is just that type of philosophy—a young nurse who has gained experience and now is called to continue her education and share her knowledge by coaching and mentoring students in a clinical instructor role.

**Exhibit 6.2**  Philosophy and Goals:
Jeana Dunn, BSN, RN

I believe that each individual is a unique being with physical, psychological, social, and spiritual needs. Francis Marion University's Department of Nursing has a philosophy that focuses on caring for the entire patient. This requires one to be a competent nurse who knows what to do at crucial times with an ability to critically think. It also necessitates being committed not only to the profession, but to those for whom we serve on a daily basis. Also of importance

*Continued*

**Exhibit 6.2**  *Continued*

to our philosophical framework is the concept of caring, which is exhibited by showing concern and providing compassionate care for others. One crucial aspect of caring for others is possessing the quality of empathy. This involves being able to truly care for others by understanding their feelings and identifying with them as an individual being. As a student nurse, one of my goals has been to truly understand the role of a professional nurse, and the philosophy of our nursing department has helped to mold me into the person that I am today; therefore, I will always keep this philosophy in my heart as a guiding light.

There is much more to nursing than solely the paperwork and hands-on, task-related work. The concepts of caring, commitment, and competence are all vital components of any nurse, and they form the foundation for my philosophy. I now have a better understanding of the meta-paradigm of health, human beings, nursing, and the environment. I am also more culturally competent, as much of my course work has instructed me on the variations of cultures around the world, as well as the differences among ethnicities. Various clinical and community service opportunities have opened my eyes to the realities of present day health care, and to the fact that not all people can afford the opportunities to receive adequate care without assistance from volunteer organizations. My personal philosophy aligns with the philosophy of Dr. Jean Watson's premise, which recognizes nursing as both a philosophical and scientific approach to caring for all those who

*Continued*

**Exhibit 6.2** *Continued*

seek health care, disease prevention and management, health promotion, and education. Watson's Ten Carative Factors encompass the qualities that are essential in establishing therapeutic communication and relationships between the patient and the nurse. I realize that caring can make a huge difference in the therapeutic relationship of the nurse and patient, and it also contains a healing factor for patients, as they are able to experience genuine care that is focused specifically on them as a unique individual.

During my nursing career, I will base my principles on this foundational basis, which will assist me in providing quality, non-judgmental, competent care to all that I come in contact with. I will take these experiences and apply them to my nursing practices by focusing on caring for the patient holistically. The care that nurses have the ability to provide to patients is irreplaceable, and no patient should be faced with a situation in which the "care" that they receive is any less than therapeutic, patient-centered, holistic care. I will always keep these early experiences in mind, and will refer to them when times are challenging or when I see another nurse struggling and in need of encouragement. Nursing is my way of giving back to society; giving of myself gives me peace of mind and spirit, and I have a goal of providing the best of care to all I come in contact with. I have found there is far more to healing than medicine alone. The ability to truly show a person that you care involves interacting with that person

*Continued*

**Exhibit 6.2**  *Continued*

on a spiritual level. Compassionate nursing provides competent, individualized care for the patient, remembering that healing is impacted by true quality care, which is solely focused on that individual's needs. Without this therapeutic environment, complete healing is inhibited. In conclusion, my experience in Francis Marion University's nursing program has been full of matchless learning experiences and cherished memories. I know that I will never forget these experiences, and they are truly the building blocks of my future career. I realize that my individual success will depend solely on my individual perseverance and dedication. I can honestly say that with such experiences behind me and my entire future before me, I have received training and education that will assist me in becoming a competent, confident nurse.

My goals for nursing included first receiving a job as a registered nurse on a general medical-surgical hospital floor. After spending time on a general medical-surgical floor to practice my nursing skills, I acquired a position as an obstetrical nurse. Now, I aspire to go back to further my education by getting my nurse practitioner degree and working as a clinical instructor for undergraduate nursing students. I feel I have gained experience and insight and can offer them the guidance they need to progress from novice to proficient student nurses.

## TEACHING RESPONSIBILITY

The next section of *Part 2: Teaching* of your academic portfolio should include your teaching responsibilities so the reviewers know exactly what you teach, how often, and to how many learners (Morin, 2006). Some authors call this section along with the teaching philosophy "the reflective analysis" part. It should provide the reviewers with:

- Number of clinical/or theory credits
- Level of the course in the program
- Number of students (Appling, Naumann, & Berk, 2001)

This can be done simply with an introductory statement and a clearly organized table as shown in Table 6.1. An introductory statement should explain how the courses you teach fit into the overall curriculum (Melland & Volden, 1996).

## TEACHING DIMENSIONS

In the narrative section that follows your teaching philosophy and the teaching responsibility chart, you should clearly demonstrate the following points:

- Your teaching design
- Your enactment of teaching
- The results of your teaching (Corry & Timmons, 2009)

Exhibit 6.3 demonstrates how to normatively include the above points in the paragraphs about your teaching:

**TABLE 6.1** Summary of Teaching Responsibility

| Semester/<br>Quarter | Course # | Course<br>Title | Credits | Class<br>Hours | Lab<br>Hours | Number of<br>Students<br>Enrolled |
|---|---|---|---|---|---|---|
| Sp 2010 | NURS 303 | Women's Health | 6 | 3 | 9 | 64 |
| Fall 2010 | NURS 303 | Women's Health | 6 | 3 | 9 | 64 |
| Fall 2010 | GEN 407 | Women & Society | 3 | 3 | 0 | 24 |
| Sp 2011 | NURS 502 | Nursing Theory | 3 | 3 | 0 | 15 |
| Sp 2011 | NURS 333 | Professional Concepts | 3 | 3 | 0 | 64 |
| Sp 2011 | UNIV 100 | Freshmen Seminar | 3 | 3 | 0 | 82 |
| Total for academic year 2010–2011 | | | 18 | 15 | 9 | 249 |

**Exhibit 6.3** Teaching Dimensions

Header: Undergraduate teaching

During my career at _____ I have taught all levels of nursing students. I am passionate about teaching undergraduate women's health and have done so twice (Spring 2009 and Fall 2010). My student's evaluations for the first time I taught the course are included in the Appendix _____. This course was team taught and I learned a tremendous amount from the course leader about teaching large classes. Although most of the content of this important junior-level clinical course was taught by lecture, I integrated the use of discussion of pre-made case studies (Appendix _____). The active learning experiences were structured to simulate real clinical experiences. The student evaluations of the course were favorable (Appendix _____), but indicated that I covered content too fast. A peer evaluation of my teaching in this course also suggested I decrease the amount of content on each PowerPoint® slide in order to slow the pace. After reflecting on these evaluations, I altered my classroom techniques by decreasing the amount of information I had on each PowerPoint and providing a class plan or organization outline in the beginning of each class. I also used the ARS (automated response system) for each class to increase the instructiveness appropriate to large groups. These altered classroom techniques were well-received by both learners and peer evaluators as shown in the evaluations after the second time I taught Women's Health (Appendix _____).

*Continued*

**Exhibit 6.3**  *Continued*

Below is the grade distribution (Exhibit 6.4) for both times I taught the Women's Health Course, which is an important clinical course in the nursing student's junior year. As you can see from the grade distribution, I have maintained course rigor. It is a course that has three lecture hours and nine clinical hours a week. At this point in their educational career, learners must be able to integrate concepts from fundamental and medical surgical nursing as well as personal interactions skills from mental health nursing. Learners must pass both the clinical and didactic portions of the course in order to advance in the curriculum to the next clinical course.

**Exhibit 6.4**

Class ($N$ = 64) GPA Sp 2010 (light columns) = 2.75
Class ($N$ = 64) GPA Fall 2010 (dark columns) = 2.35

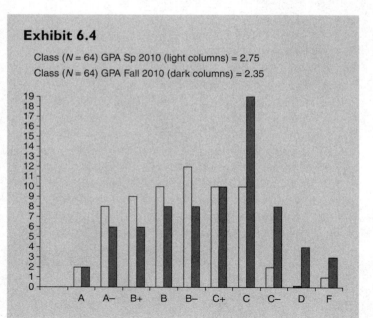

This example of a narrative paragraph demonstrates that key teaching points as outlined by Corry and Timmons (2009) were addressed. How it was taught (teaching design and enactment) is included (PowerPoint, discussion, case studies, ARS), and evidence of these methods should be reflected in the course syllabus. The narrative paragraph also included how it was received or evaluated and evidence is included in the appendices, both learner and peer.

## OTHER IMPORTANT POINTS ABOUT YOUR TEACHING NARRATIVE

Other models of exactly what to include under the teaching part of your portfolio have been offered by other authors. Urbach (1992) states an academic portfolio should include:

- How one teaches
- Changes in one's teaching
- Rigor of one's academic standards
- Student's impression of one's teaching
- How your colleagues assess your teaching

═══════════════════════════*FAST FACTS in a NUTSHELL*

When crafted carefully and concisely, your narrative can accomplish the overarching purpose of the academic portfolio: It can showcase your accomplishments in teaching scholarship, show personal and professional development, and explain to other academics specifics about nursing education.

## CONTINUING WITH YOUR PERSONAL STATEMENT ABOUT TEACHING SCHOLARSHIP

After you describe the courses you have been involved in using a model that explains what you teach, how you teach, and the outcomes of your teaching, you may want to include other information about your teaching scholarship. Listed are some ideas or topics that are appropriate to include in this section:

- New courses you have developed
- Teaching awards and recognitions (Oermann, 1999)
- Program development
- Use of innovative technology to enhance teaching
- Course revision
- Professional development (Francis Marion University, 2011)

Exhibits 6.5 and 6.6 are other examples of a Teaching Section of a personal statement used successfully for promotion from instructor to assistant professor by Dr. Rhonda Brogdon.

**Exhibit 6.5**   Teaching Statement: Dr. Rhonda Brogdon

Since 2005, I have received stellar evaluations from my students and my Department Chair regarding my teaching. I have been flexible and have taught numerous different courses depending on departmental need. I have been a course coordinator for Fundamentals/Adult Health I (NURS 304) and was also a clinical instructor for the course. This was an

*Continued*

**Exhibit 6.5**  *Continued*

extremely important course in our curriculum since
it lays the foundation for all the students' clinical
experiences. This course also required an extensive
orientation and entrance nursing math exam prior to
its start; I coordinated both events.

In 2007, I was a guest lecturer in Health Assessment
(NURS 301) and was an assistant course coordinator and lab instructor. I continue to work as a lab
instructor and frequently guest lecture. Thorough
physical assessment skills are currently recognized
as an important variable in the clinical area in order
to reduce the incidences of failure-to-rescue. I have
also was a guest lecturer in Population Focused
Nursing (NURS 402) and also taught clinical for
the course. This course provided students about the
importance of community involvement and clinical
understandings of the health and illness experiences
of individuals and families within the area and global
populations. I coordinated a lab day experiences for
students in NURS 402 to review techniques for accurate intramuscular injections for their experience in
the health department for flu season injections.

Currently, I teach Nursing Research in Practice
(NURS 306). Nursing research is one of the more
difficult courses for undergraduate nursing students
because it deals with abstract concepts as opposed
to clinical processes. It is important that the students have a firm foundation in nursing research in
order to function in the evidence-based health care
environment of today. Since my research course has
been such a success with the traditional students,

*Continued*

**Exhibit 6.5**   *Continued*

I have been asked to teach the RN-to-BSN students in spring of 2011. I have volunteered to become course coordinator of Health Assessment during week six of the fall 2010 semester due to an abrupt resignation of a faculty member. I am comfortable teaching online as well as in the classroom.

**Exhibit 6.6**   Teaching Statement:
             Dr. Rosemary Fliszar

I believe that students need to be engaged in the learning process and that my role as a faculty member is to facilitate that learning through a variety of activities. Since all of the students in the RN-BSN program have completed their initial education at either a Community College (ADN) or diploma program (such as that offered at Reading Hospital School of Nursing) and have passed the RN licensing exam (NCLEX), I feel it is important to build upon the knowledge, experience, and skills which they have accumulated in their initial program and as a working RN. The students in the Master's program also are working RNs in a variety of settings and I use strategies in those courses to build upon their experiences and teach them the theoretical principles related to the role of the nurse educator. Therefore, I employ principles of adult learning as espoused by Knowle's Adult Learning Theory. Active involvement in the classroom and outside activities

*Continued*

**Exhibit 6.6**   *Continued*

is essential to promote learning, and I employ as
many active strategies as possible in each of my
courses. I also recognize that students have different learning styles as outlined in Gardner's Theory
of Multiple Intelligences, so I use multiple methods
in the classroom and online courses to meet the
needs of students who learn by various methods of
intelligence, such as visual/spatial, kinesthetic, etc.
I engage students based on these theories through a
variety of different learning activities. I often use the
Socratic method in class to draw upon their previous knowledge, and employ this same method in my
online courses by posting questions on the discussion board on Blackboard or D2L. I encourage open
dialogue in my classes so students can share their
experiences related to the topics being discussed
in class. I use the internet to supplement material
being presented; for example, I have shown a music
video to the graduate students which focuses on an
elderly man expressing his thoughts about growing old gracefully. Students are then asked to discuss what types of courses this video could be used
in and how it reinforces learning. In several of my
courses, especially those with a clinical component
or the practicum, students write journals discussing
their experiences and what they have learned. These
activities allow the student to reflect on their experiences and promote active learning.

Nurses must remain current in their field as
health care changes rapidly. Since nursing is a

*Continued*

**Exhibit 6.6**  *Continued*

profession, nurses must also meet the ideals set forth in a profession, such as lifelong learning. A scholarly paper is required in all of my courses in both the undergraduate and graduate programs. The papers require students to conduct a literature review from professional journals and include articles that are evidence based. I impress upon the students the importance of making decisions in their delivery of care to individuals or in their teaching activities based upon sound theoretical and proven research.

In courses offered in the classroom setting students do presentations on selected topics as assigned in each course. I encourage them to use a variety of activities when doing these projects. Students who are enrolled in the courses online are held to similar expectations as those in the classroom. They do their presentations through podcasting on Blackboard or D2L, and their classmates listen to the podcasts and do peer evaluations as is done in the face-to-face classroom setting. I have included in my documents directives for the various activities required in each of my courses.

I have many years of experience working in nursing as well as education, and I share some of my experiences with students to help them better understand the concepts being presented. Many times students stay after class, stop by my office, or call me for further discussion. I maintain an open door policy and serve as a resource to my students.

## EVIDENCE TO SUPPORT THE TEACHING SECTION OF YOUR PERSONAL STATEMENT

### *FAST FACTS in a NUTSHELL*

The evidence (artifacts) that you include directly support statements you make in your personal statement.

Evidence may include the following items:

- Course syllabi
- Class handouts
- Use of technology
- Samples of learners' work
- Exam accomplishments (class or standardized testing)
- Clinical evaluations of students
- Student evaluations of class and educator trended over time
- Peer evaluations
- Videotapes of teaching (Appling et al., 2001)
- Sample instructional material (Oermann, 1999)
- Evaluation rubrics
- Care plans
- Integration of service learning into course
- Letters from students or alumni addressing your teaching effectiveness (Melland & Volden, 1996)

You may have examples of other evidence that demonstrates your teaching scholarship; thus, this list presents suggestions and is not all inclusive.

========================================*FAST FACTS in a NUTSHELL*

Do not forget that each portfolio is individual to the
nurse educator!

## SUMMARY

*Part 2: Teaching* of your personal statement follows your
preface. Part 2 is usually subdivided into a narrative section that includes your teaching philosophy, teaching
responsibilities, and teaching scholarship. It is important
to describe how you teach, what the outcomes of your
teaching are, and how you reflect and appraise those outcomes. The next chapter will discuss the scholarship of
research and publishing.

========================================*FAST FACTS in a NUTSHELL*

Ongoing outline of your academic portfolio:
1. Part 1: Preface/Abstract (approximately 1
   page)
2. Part 1: Teaching (3–6 pages)
3. Teaching Philosophy (1 page of the 3 to 6
   pages)
4. Teaching Responsibilities
5. Narrative About Teaching Scholarship

# 7

## How to Showcase Your Research and/or Scholarship

## INTRODUCTION

This chapter will focus on the scholarship of research (Part 3 of your academic portfolio) or what the Boyer (1990) model of scholarship would refer to as "discovery." Not all nurse educators are in a research intensive university so they may not have to produce original research. Many nurse educators in positions that expect the discovery of new knowledge must write grants to support their research activity, so grant writing would also be included in this section. Regardless of the type of institution in which a nurse educator is a faculty member, all nurse educators use research to promote their scholarship of teaching. By using up-to-date evidence in educational practice you are an important consumer of research. Many times your course outcome data (grades, evaluations, and informal feedback) inform you of the effectiveness of your educational interventions that are based on evidence. This is valuable information and if it has not been included in your Part 2: Teaching section of your personal statement, then

> *it should be include here in* Part 3: Research and/or Scholarship *section. Note that in this section "scholarship" is used differently than it was in Chapter 1 where it describes a general condition of inquiry. Here scholarship is used as the academic attainment of the scholar (Dictionary.com, 2011) in reference to publications. In academia, the word scholarship is often interchanged to mean authored work and many academics consider publication as a goal of scholarship.*

At the end of this chapter, the nurse educator will be able to:

1. Distinguish between research activity and the scholarship of publication.
2. Understand the interrelatedness of the two types of scholarship.
3. Describe the interrelatedness of the scholarship of publications with that of teaching.

## RESEARCH

Grant writing to obtain the financial resources to carry out research is included in this section. Even if the grant or award is small and internal (given by your own institution), it is significant and should be included because the process to obtain it was competitive to some extent. All research, whether educational or clinical, or in progress or completed during your years at the institution, should be included. If you are developing a portfolio in order to be hired, then previous research should be included. Any role that you have had on a research project should be included in your portfolio with an accurate description of your role. Common roles in research include:

- Principal Investigator (PI): This is the person who is responsible for the research project.

- Program or Project Director (PD): This is similar to a PI but may also be in charge of monies to run an educational program.
- Co-Investigator (Co-I): This is the person who, with the PI, helps complete the research and is also responsible for proper use of the money awarded by a grant.
- Consultant: This is the person who provides information or services to the PI to assist with the research (an example is a statistician).
- Human Subject: This is the person the research is being done to and is sometimes called the participant.
- Key Personnel: These are people who contribute to the research process and may include the PI, Co-I, and others working on the research (National Institutes of Health [NIH], 2011).
- Data Collector: This is a person who helps collect research data and sometimes enters it into a data base for the researchers.

═══════════════════════════*FAST FACTS in a NUTSHELL*

For an academic portfolio with a concentration on research, Part 3 may be five or six pages long; for institutions that are not research intensive, this section may be two to three pages in length.

Peterson and Sandholtz (2005) discuss including any collaborative grant writing as a valuable activity, whether or not funding was awarded. However, it is more important to list grants and research that have been funded. Listing grants and research projects that have been denied funding may not be advantageous if seeking advancement in an institution that expects successful funding, but it may be done to demonstrate effort toward obtaining a grant, as is illustrated in Exhibit 7.1.

**Exhibit 7.1**    My Mid-Point Academic Portfolio on Research and Scholarship

Fifty percent of my position was allocated to research. Because I have clinical expertise in both women's health and neonatal care, I have two distinct and exciting areas of research and scholarship.

Decisional Science in Women's Health

In 2006, I published my concept analysis on my developing practice theory, "The Wittmann-Price Theory of Emancipated Decision-Making in Women's Healthcare." The theory was retroductively formulated based on 30 years of direct clinical care to mothers and infants. I studied the concepts contained in my theory in order to meet my dissertation requirements and found that an emancipated decision was positively and significantly related to decisional satisfaction. Shortly after graduation, I published the results of my dissertation. That study was cited three times as a positive mechanism to better understand gender specific decision making. After graduation in May of 2006, I studied my practice theory (unfunded) a second time with a different clinical exemplar to compare results. The second study verified the results of the first study and was published in 2008. After I was hired, I studied my practice theory a third time with funds from a chapter of Sigma Theta Tao International. The third study

*Continued*

**Exhibit 7.1**  *Continued*

refined the concepts and the instrument. Publication of the third study has been accepted and the instrument development manuscript has been submitted. One of the limitations of all three studies was that they were done with a homogeneous population. My current clinical contacts will provide me the opportunity to increase population diversity in order to be able to investigate decisional science for more women. I have submitted several grants to continue the study of EDM and they are listed in Table 7.1.

TABLE 7.1   Grant Submission Pertaining to Decisional Science

| Date | Sponsor | Title | Outcome |
|------|---------|-------|---------|
| Sept 2007 | STTI Nu Eta | Exploring Emancipated Decision Making About Delivery Options in Women's Healthcare. | Funded $1000 |
| May 2008 | ANF (American Nurses Foundation) | The Effect of Emancipated Decision Making on 3-Month Infant Feeding Follow-Up Rates | Denied with encouragement to resubmit |
| Oct 2008 | GRANT 00520712 NIH PA-08–064 | Evaluation of Decision Aids for a Single-Event Intervention for Breast Cancer | Unscored |
| March 2009 | ONS (Oncology Nurse Society Grant) | Decision Making for Adjuvant Therapy in Women Diagnosed With Breast Cancer | Unfunded |
| April 2009 | GRANT NIH | Stimulus Grant: Using a Predictive Model for Decisional Follow-Through in Women's Healthcare | Pending |
| May 2009 | ANF Resubmission | The Effect of Emancipated Decision Making on 3-Month Infant Feeding Follow-Up Rates | Pending |

The first NIH grant summary from October of 2008 was not encouraging, and I lacked the expertise in cancer care. The Stimulus grant, although

*Continued*

**Exhibit 7.1**   *Continued*

unfunded, had comments that did encourage me to
further develop a study to use my own theoretical
framework. The comments from the NIH reviewers
on the investigator item all spoke to my expertise in
this area and regarded it as a strength. I am working
on a resubmission for October of 2009. It is an RO3
on women's decision making using my theory to pre-
dict follow-through on breastfeeding, for one of the
*Healthy People 2010* initiatives.

The Wittmann-Price Theory has been presented
locally, nationally, and internationally as noted in
Table 7.2. I was also accepted to present my third
study in Cancun, Mexico, in July of 2009, at the
International Research Conference of Sigma Theta
Tao International but I was unable to attend.

TABLE 7.2    **Presentations of the Wittmann-Price
Emancipated Decision Making in
Women's Healthcare Theory**

| Date | Outcome |
|---|---|
| *International Conferences* July 2006 | **Wittmann-Price, R. A.** *Emancipated Decision Making in Women's Healthcare.* STTI Evidence-Based Practice, Montreal, Canada |
| *National Conferences* Feb 2009 | **Wittmann-Price, R. A.** *Emancipated Decision Making in Women's Healthcare About Delivery Choice.* Women's Health Conference, Atlantic City, New Jersey |
| Feb 2008 | **Wittmann-Price, R. A.** *Emancipated Decision Making in Women's Healthcare.* 32nd Annual Planned Parenthood Federation of American and Drexel University, Women's Health Conference, Atlantic City, New Jersey |

*Continued*

**Exhibit 7.1**  *Continued*

Developmental Care of the Preterm Infant

My second research interest, neurodevelopment of the preterm infant, has been served through my position. Our university's association with a major children's hospital provides a tremendous opportunity for me to study the effects of the environment on the preterm infant. I participated in a study to decrease environmental noise in the neonatal intensive care unit (NICU) and have just finished a study using cyclic light to decrease length of stay, which has been submitted for publication. I submitted a grant (RO3) to study olfactory stimulation; although it was not scored, my consultant believes it can be rectified and resubmitted. This will be done in the form of a 2010 *NIH Director's New Innovator Award Program (DP2) for 2–26–09*. This research endeavor is an extension of a pilot study done in France that showed robust results using vanillin scent to decrease apnea of prematurity (AOP). A list of my grants submitted to study the preterm newborn are listed in Table 7.3.

**TABLE 7.3   Grants Submitted to Study Preterm Infant Neurodevelopment**

| Date | Sponsor | Title | Outcome |
|---|---|---|---|
| Nov 2008 | AWHONN (Association of Women's Health, Obstetrics and Neonatal Nurses) | The Relationship of Olfactory Stimulation on Apnea of Prematurity | Unfunded |
| Oct 2008 | PA-06–180 NIH | The Relationship of Olfactory Stimulation on Apnea of Prematurity | Unfunded |
| May 27, 2009 | March of Dimes | Collaborative Effort for Decrease of Preterm Births in Philadelphia | Pending |

*Continued*

**Exhibit 7.1**  *Continued*

Unfortunately, it has taken 2 years to fine tune the grant submission because I did not have a post-doctorate fellowship. I have learned a tremendous amount during the past 2 years and feel my network in decisional science is expanding. I am confident that I am getting close to funding and am willing to continue trying to the best of my ability.

## PUBLICATIONS AND PRESENTATIONS

As you can determine from the exhibits in this chapter, publications and presentations are an expected consequence of research. Once a topic is studied, it is our professional responsibility to disseminate the results to increase the knowledge base of nursing science.

$$\equiv FAST\ FACTS\ in\ a\ NUTSHELL$$

Data-driven publications are well respected but they are not the only publications needed by and for nurse educators.

Any publication space contributed to you should be included on your Curriculum Vitae. Examples of your best publications can be included in your appendices. "Best" can be interpreted in many different ways: It can mean your publications in the highest impact journals (journals in a discipline that are most read and cited), or those in journals with a vast readership (an example would be *American Journal of Nursing*).

Peer-reviewed publications should be distinguished from invited publications. Articles about nursing education itself and innovative teaching strategies are a wonderful integration of teaching scholarship with publication. Also include any book chapters that you may have written or contributed to, and of course any books you may have written.

===*FAST FACTS in a NUTSHELL*

It is not usual to list manuscripts that were submitted and rejected or that are under review, but you can list manuscripts submitted that have been accepted and have not yet been published as "in press."

## PRESENTATIONS

In order to be accepted for a presentation, a nurse educator must establish an expertise in an area and submit an abstract about that expertise. Presentations are usually listed by regional, national, and international categories. Do not forget to include the fact that you may have given multiple regional presentations to area practice partners! Those presentations are not only scholarship but are also service if they are unpaid. As before, you should distinguish between peer-reviewed and invited presentations: Both are prestigious, but they are different.

## EVIDENCE TO SUPPORT THE RESEARCH AND/OR SCHOLARSHIP SECTION OF YOUR PERSONAL STATEMENT

Some of the evidence that you may want to include to support the claims you have made in this section of your portfolio can be selected items from the following:

- Articles
- Books
- Book chapters
- Editorials
- Reviews
- Learning modules
- E-learning activities
- Presentation abstracts
- Consultation write-ups
- Editing
- Grants (Peterson & Sandholtz, 2005)

## SUMMARY

This chapter distinguished between research activity and scholarship in the form of publications and presentations, but helped you to recognize how teaching, research, and publications can also be very interrelated. This chapter also emphasized that different types of institutions will view these scholarships with different weighted perspectives during an evaluation process. The next chapter will discuss *Part 4: Service.*

## *FAST FACTS in a NUTSHELL*

Ongoing outline of your academic portfolio:

1. Part 1: Preface/Abstract (approximately 1 page)
2. Part 2: Teaching (3–6 pages)
   a. Teaching Philosophy (1 page of the 3 to 6 pages)
   b. Teaching Responsibilities
   c. Narrative About Teaching Scholarship
3. Part 3: Research and/or Scholarship (2–6 pages)
   a. Research Activities
   b. Publications and Presentations

# 8

## How to Showcase Your Service

### INTRODUCTION

*This chapter will discuss service. Service is expected of professionals in academic positions. It is not just about what we as nurse educations get from a system, but also what we give back. This is just a natural part of being a professional and being passionate about your discipline and calling as an educator.*

At the end of this chapter, the nurse educator will be able to:

1. Describe three types of professional service.
2. Distinguish between departmental and university service.
3. Understand what type of community service is appropriate to include.

## TYPES OF SERVICE

All institutions expect professional service to some varying degree. Service is the most widely defined of the scholarships but is basically divided into three types:

- Service to the department
- Service to the institution
- Service to the community

This section—*Part 4: Service*—of your academic portfolio is usually about two to three pages in length; most portfolios do take at least two pages to describe service.

## Service to the Department

Your service to your nursing educational unit is very important. Although there is an administrator in every department, academic departments should be governed by faculty. Faculty should own the curriculum and make the decisions about the educational content to uphold faculty governance. We all know that it is not acceptable for just some members of the faculty to contribute; all must contribute to ensure the success of the team and the accomplishment of the mission. Therefore, your departmental contributions are most important and can encompass a wide range of activities. Some of those activities are:

- Committee membership
- Student advising
- Service-learning activities
- Mentorship of novice faculty
- Steering committees
- Interviewing faculty candidates
- Supporting students at scholarship dinners
- Administrative coverage
- Peer-reviewing courses

- Assisting in accreditation preparation
- Guest lecturing
- Covering another faculty member's responsibilities, if needed
- Attending alumni functions
- Participating in departmental open houses
- Involvement in student activities
- Advisor for student clubs
- Advisor for social organizations
- Assisting in student activities

This is not an exhaustive list. Departmental service is something that you must reflect upon almost on a day-to-day basis.

=======================*FAST FACTS in a NUTSHELL*

If it is not an activity for which you are receiving course credit or compensation and if it is outside of the normal day-to-day responsibilities described in your job description, then it very well may be departmental service and should be noted.

## Institutional Service

Besides departmental service, institutional service is also important for the same reasons—to ensure that the mission of the institution is being carried out and to ensure faculty governance. There are many ways tenured and non-tenured faculty can participate. University committees are the obvious place where service is recognized but participating in other activities not only assists the institution to function efficiently, but also showcases yourself and nursing. Some of these activities may include:

- Participating in university or college open houses
- Interviewing incoming freshman for scholarships
- Assisting with ad hoc committees or task forces
- Being present at general faculty meetings to vote
- Participating in fund raising activities
- Assisting with general freshman orientation
- Becoming a faculty workgroup or task force member
- Serving as program director (Francis Marion University, 2011).

Again, this is not an exhaustive list and each institution will have different activities that are open to faculty.

## *FAST FACTS in a NUTSHELL*

One of the worst scenarios that can happen to a person going for tenure or promotion is for the committee members not being able to put a face to the name.

## Community Service

Community service can also be called professional service. It is those activities that are related to nursing but not to the university or department. These services may include:

- Board memberships for health care-related institutions
- Volunteer clinical service
- Membership in national or international nursing committees

- Precepting nurse educator students from other institutions
- Providing health care consultation to outsider groups without accepting compensation
- Developing a parish nursing organization
- Participating in an emergency response system for bioterrorism
- Volunteering as a school or camp nurse

The common thread among community service activities is they are health care related and are unpaid. Other community service such as Girl Scout Troop leader is wonderful, but they are not related to the profession of nursing and therefore should not be listed. Exhibits 8.1 and 8.2 are examples of a *Part 4: Service* section of a personal statement for an academic portfolio.

---

**Exhibit 8.1**  Service

I have been involved in service activities on the departmental, college, and community level. My departmental governance includes guest lecturing, proctoring two- and three-hour midterm and final exams, monitoring at events (graduation ceremonies), and presenting at open houses, both undergraduate and doctoral, which are hosted from 4 to 6 p.m. once a month. I also participate in committee activities.

   I am a member of the undergraduate nursing curriculum committee. I have developed a tutorial for new faculty to assist them to evaluate test questions and develop a syllabus. I have contributed to revising and writing new undergraduate level objectives

*Continued*

**Exhibit 8.1**  *Continued*

and defining program outcomes. The task of leveling the objectives involves a team that dedicates a half-day workshop to the task. The objectives are still being refined; I am an active member of the group and we continue to meet on a monthly basis.

Last year I served on the student conduct committee. That committee met frequently—approximately eight times during the year—in order to hear incidents on a spontaneous time frame to discuss the outcome of students' grievances. There were approximately three cases that needed the guidance of the committee and the nature of the cases prompted the committee to develop guidelines. I assisted with the development of those guidelines and, on occasion, recorded the minutes and assisted in the development of by-laws.

I am on the doctoral admissions committee and evaluate every applicant; there are approximately 20 applications each year. When an application is complete, the administrative assistant forwards the package and I need to assess the qualifications of the candidate within 48 hours, which can be completed accurately in approximately one hour. The other role I have on that committee is pre-interviews. Occasionally we receive information about a candidate who may have a low Graduate Entrance Exam (GRE) score. The committee chair and I meet with the candidate and decipher if the score was an actual assessment of ability or if it was a matter of an unexplained situation. We have met three candidates thus far and all have had extraordinary circumstances and have been advised to retake the GRE.

*Continued*

**Exhibit 8.1**  *Continued*

I also administratively covered the program when the administrator was out of town. I serve as the second reader for a current dissertation candidate who will defend May 1, 2010, and have been a contributing member of the audience to two dissertation presentations and the fifth reader for another.

On the university level, in January of 2009 I was on a per-invitation interview committee to choose a faculty member for the School of Technology. We interviewed two people and met several times to discuss the qualifications needed for the position, as well as to evaluate the comparative qualifications of the interviewed candidates.

I assisted with Magnet symposia and presented research activity. There have been hospital-wide symposia each spring and fall for the past 2 years that included presentations in one of the larger auditoriums. In the previous two symposia I presented the work of the Nursing Research Council using a PowerPoint presentation. In the second symposium, I introduced the nurses to clicker technology. Plans for the upcoming symposium include the setting up of an informational table.

I am on a dissertation committee by request from a doctoral student from Widener University who is a studying a women's health issue. I have given her feedback on her proposal thus far and am awaiting revisions.

I also work every Wednesday from 5 to 8 p.m. on a volunteer basis at the Chinatown clinic. I perform intake histories of patients, provide physical assessments, triage, advocate, and health teach. It is a

*Continued*

**Exhibit 8.1**  *Continued*

rewarding experience that sometimes includes supporting the learning experiences of the RN to BSN students and medical students who are working in the clinic during my volunteer hours.

I participate in the "Race for Hope" every fall to fundraise for brain cancer research. In my home community, I am a member of the Emergency Medical System and I tutor local students who need assistance to pass their RN licensure exam.

**Exhibit 8.2**  From Dr. Rosemary Fliszar's Section Describing Her Service to the Nursing Profession

Part 4: Evidence of Service and Contribution to the University and/or Community

A. Quality of Participation in Program, Department, College, and University Committees

*Membership on University Committees*

| 2009–Present | Center for the Enhancement of Teaching Advisory Council |
| 2008–Present | Graduate Council Member—Policy Committee |
| 2007–2009 | Commission on Human Diversity |

*Continued*

**Exhibit 8.2**   *Continued*

| | |
|---|---|
| 2007–2008; 2009 | University Curriculum Committee (Spring 2009: Substituted as the Graduate Council representative for a member who was on sabbatical) |
| 2007–2007 | University Senate, Fall of 2007 (Substituted for department representative who was unable to attend due to class conflict) |
| 2010–Present | Appointed by the nursing faculty to serve as the department representative to the Senate effective 11–6–10 |
| 2006–2007 | APSCUF |

*Membership on College Committees*

| | |
|---|---|
| 2007–2008 | College of Liberal Arts and Sciences Curriculum Committee |

*Membership on Committees/Responsibilities in Nursing Department*

| | |
|---|---|
| 2006–Present | Nursing Faculty Organization |
| 2006–Present | PET Committee |
| 2006–Present | Program Evaluation Committee |
| 2006–Present | Policies/By-laws Committee |
| 2006–2009 | Curriculum Committee; Chairperson, 2006–2007 |

*Continued*

**Exhibit 8.2**  *Continued*

| | |
|---|---|
| 2007–2007 | Chair, Faculty Search Committee (Spring and Fall, 2007) |
| 2008–2009 | Chair, Faculty Search Committee |
| 2008–Present | Graduate Committee; Chairperson, 2008–Present |
| 2008–Present | MSN Coordinator |
| 2009–2010 | Team Leader and Member, NLNAC Self-Study Report Committee |

### B. Development of New Courses

In fall of 2009, the Nursing Department Graduate Committee recommended revision of the current Nurse Educator track in the MSN program, and the addition of a Clinical Nurse Leader track to the program. As a result I developed several new courses for the Nurse Educator track, which were approved by UCC. The syllabi for these courses are included as part of this application. I also revised several courses in the MSN program as part of this revision and those syllabi are also included in the packet. Due to the recent decision by Administration to place the MSN program in moratorium, the new curriculum has not been put into place. Therefore the new graduate courses will not be implemented at this time; however, the revised graduate courses have been implemented.

*New Graduate Courses Developed*

| | |
|---|---|
| NUR 515 | Technology in Nursing Education and Practice |
| NUR 592 | Role of the Nurse Educator |

*Continued*

**Exhibit 8.2** *Continued*

| | |
|---|---|
| NUR 593 | Nursing Education Immersion II |
| NUR 594 | Nurse Educator Capstone Seminar |

*Graduate Courses Revised*

| | |
|---|---|
| NUR 505 | Strategies in Adult Education (Formerly NUR 490) |
| NUR 540 | Curriculum and Instructional Design |

A full discussion of courses that I developed and taught or currently teach is included under "Scholarly Growth—Development of Experimental Programs and Innovative Teaching Strategies."

### C. Assist Other Faculty Members in the Use of Distance Education Technology

On numerous occasions I have worked with faculty in the Nursing Department to assist them in using the online learning platforms, such as Blackboard. I have shown two faculty members how to set up the grade book. I developed a handout on how to produce and post a Podcast on Blackboard and have shared this with all faculty in the Nursing Department. I assisted a faculty member in conducting a live class in the online classroom; I taught another faculty member how to use the Chat room on Blackboard and D2L to hold online office hours. I helped several faculty members set up an account on SKYPE and demonstrated how to use it for class and conferences.

*Continued*

**Exhibit 8.2**  *Continued*

D. Participate in University-Wide Colloquia

I have attended several workshops sponsored by Kutztown University and the Center for the Enhancement of Teaching. I also attend presentations on topics that assist me in using the online learning platforms, Blackboard and now D2L, with Will Jefferson. Certificates of attendance are found in Binder #2. I have attended the following colloquia/workshops:

- "Ebrary at Kutztown University Workshop," April 29, 2010. Sponsored by the Kutztown University Center for the Enhancement of Teaching
- "Meeting the Challenges of the Writing Intensive Classroom," presented by Amy Lynch-Biniek, January 12, 2010
- "Basics of Wimba Classroom Workshop," Spring 2009. Sponsored by Kutztown University Center for the Enhancement of Teaching
- "Introduction to Instant Survey Workshop," Fall 2008. Sponsored by Kutztown University Center for the Enhancement of Teaching

E. Advisor to Student Organizations

In the 2006–2007 and 2007–2008 academic years, I served as Faculty Advisor to the Xi Omega Chapter, Sigma Theta Tau. Sigma Theta Tau is the International Nursing Honor Society, and Xi Omega is the chapter at Kutztown University. Membership into the Society is based on academic achievement and is selective. Xi Omega offers a research night each year as part of their programming, which contributes to the scholarly growth of its members.

*Continued*

**Exhibit 8.2**  *Continued*

**F. Membership in Professionally Oriented and Community-Based Organizations Related to Faculty Member's Discipline**

I am a member of several professional organizations in the discipline of nursing and nursing education, as well as on community agencies related to nursing and wellness of members of the community.

*Membership in Professional Associations*

| | |
|---|---|
| 2000–Present | Pennsylvania League for Nursing |
| 2000–Present | Pennsylvania League for Nursing Area 2 |
| 1998–Present | American Nurses Association |
| 1998–Present | Pennsylvania State Nurses Association |
| 1993–Present | Sigma Theta Tau (Nursing Honor Society): Mu Omicron Chapter, DeSales University; Xi Omega Chapter, Kutztown University |
| 1990–Present | National League for Nursing |
| 1983–Present | Alumni Association, Cedar Crest College |
| 1971–Present | Alumni Association, Lankenau Hospital School of Nursing |

In November of 2008 I was chosen to serve as the National League for Nursing (NLN) Ambassador for the nursing program at Kutztown University. "The NLN Ambassador Program engages its members in efforts to ensure that faculty and educational

*Continued*

**Exhibit 8.2**  *Continued*

leaders in all schools of nursing are kept informed about the NLN's programs, grant opportunities, and member involvement initiatives." My Ambassador responsibilities include: ensure that nursing faculty at Kutztown receive communications from the NLN; encourage faculty to participate in NLN programs; answer questions about the NLN or direct faculty to the appropriate staff; forward to the NLN issues, concerns, feedback, and suggestions from the faculty.

*Membership in Community Organizations*

2008–Present    Medical Reserve Corps,
                City of Bethlehem
2006–Present    Member, Lehigh County Office of
                Aging and Adult Services Advisory
                Council: Chairperson since 2009

Medical Reserve Corp (MRC) units are community-based, locally organized units that utilize medical professionals and others who want to donate their time and expertise to promote healthy living. Volunteers serve to supplement existing local and emergency and public health resources. The City of Bethlehem MRC is dedicated to organizing and preparing a medically related volunteer base that will assist with emergency services, public health practice, and community outreach and education.

*Continued*

**Exhibit 8.2**  *Continued*

The purpose of the Lehigh County Office of Aging and Adult Services Advisory Council is to advocate for the needs of the adult and aging community, offer suggestions for policy changes and services, and monitor existing services to be sure they meet the needs of the adult and aging population.

I served as a volunteer to enroll participants in the Cancer Prevention Study-3 for the American Cancer Society during the 2009 Relay for Life of Bethlehem, June 13, 2009. I explained the purpose of the study and interviewed potential participants to determine their eligibility to participate in the study.

I participated in the "Mass Vaccination/POD Drill" for the Bethlehem Area School District as a member of the City of Bethlehem Medical Reserve Corps, April 25, 2009. My responsibilities included interviewing people to determine their past medical and vaccination history, administering childhood vaccines to school-age children, and instructing children and their parents on possible side effects of the vaccines.

### G. Campus Presentations

I presented a session entitled *Healthy Heart* to students attending the Kutztown Preparatory Academy 2007 Summer Program on June 27, 2007.

## SUMMARY

This chapter discussed service to the profession of nursing. It described three levels of service: community, university, and department. Service to the profession is an important aspect of nursing and service learning related to educating students as global citizens is very important. The next chapter will discuss the integration of the first four parts of the personal statement.

## ═══════════════════════════════════FAST FACTS in a NUTSHELL

Ongoing outline of your academic portfolio:

1. Part 1: Preface/Abstract (approximately 1 page)
2. Part 2: Teaching (3–6 pages)
   a. Teaching Philosophy (1 page of the 3–6 pages)
   b. Teaching Responsibilities
   c. Narrative About Teaching Scholarship
3. Part 3: Research and/or Scholarship (2–6 pages)
   a. Research Activities
   b. Publications and Presentations
4. Part 4: Service (2–3 pages)
   a. Departmental
   b. Institutional
   c. Community

# 9

## How to Write an
## Integrative Summary

### INTRODUCTION

*This chapter will concentrate on the final part of your personal statement (Part 5: Integrative Summary or Review). This section "pulls it all together" by finding the links among within your scholarship of teaching, service, scholarship, and research. Seldin and Miller (2009) add two other important pieces to this section: (1) naming three things that you are especially proud of; and (2) writing three professional goals. The integrative review will be discussed in this chapter.*

At the end of this chapter, the nurse educator will be able to:

1. Describe three parts of an integrative review.
2. Craft an integrative statement that looks at both accomplishments and learned lessons.
3. Develop goals for your professional future.

## INTEGRATIVE REVIEW

The integrative review is normally 1 to 3 pages in length. It should highlight the main themes that are discussed in your academic portfolio and demonstrate how your accomplishments and goals reflect those themes. The themes can be found initially in your preface and philosophy. One way to integrate is to do a type of preliminary text analysis. Read your teaching philosophy and choose specific words that describe what you believe. In Exhibit 9.1, I have highlighted words in my teaching philosophy that are significant to me and my work.

**Exhibit 9.1**    Themes in the Teaching Philosophy

My teaching is based on the theory developed by Paulo Freire (1970) who proposed that educational institutions are powerful enough to promote an *emancipated society.* He expanded on the description of social norms that *oppress* and included the educational environment. Freire believed that oppression serves the purpose of dehumanization by producing a "culture of silence" that is exploited for political or economic gain. Because of this intellectual, emotional and psychological enslavement, the oppressed develop a "fear of freedom" (Freire, 1970, p. 36) in exchange for perceived security.

The outcome of emancipated education for any group is to *equalize power* between information giver and receiver in order to enable *free choice* and create an environment of true humanism that may extend into all social systems (Freire 1970, 1992,

*Continued*

**Exhibit 9.1**   *Continued*

1998). It was not until I read Freire's (1970) *Pedagogy of the Oppressed* that I seriously considered the social aspect as a determinate of the educational stance of people. The methodologies proposed by Freire as necessary infusions into the classroom create an equalitarian society of learning for both the educator and the learner. Freire proposes the establishment of a collaborative climate in which students take responsibility for their learning.

One of the main components of Freire's Emancipatory Education model is *reflection*, characterized by critically thinking about alternatives. Reflection can take the form of interpersonal dialogue or self-dialogue, both producing an internal awareness. Freire believed that traditional educational methods alone foster oppression because they do not encourage the reflection needed for critical thinking (Romyn, 2000). It is important to reflect on issues in order to recognize the inherent personal and social aspects. Reflection is also needed to critically think about the information gained from personal and empirical knowledge in order to synthesize it into a decision (Fahrenfort, 1987).

The next step is to find how your themes (in Exhibit 9.1, the themes are emancipated society, oppression, equalizing power, free choice, and reflection) relate to your teaching, research or scholarship, and service. An example of how themes are reflected in my teaching is how I use "extensive discussion boards and presentations" to promote reflection and how the field is equalized: "The second half of the course is a practicum, which allows me to interact with the students' and their preceptors in the field."

The themes are also reflected in my role of researcher and service in which I facilitate rather than mandate what projects are completed: "My role is to assist staff nurses in developing, implementing, and evaluating evidence-based projects." As a service, "I also work every Wednesday from 5–8 p.m. on a volunteer basis at the Chinatown clinic. I perform intake histories of patients, provide physical assessments, triage, advocate, and health teach. It is an awarding experience and at times, I assist the Drexel RN to BSN students and medical students who are in the clinic to learn." These reflect that I am providing learners with a "choice" and playing a small part in equalizing the playing field for the underserved population.

The integrative summary is where you indicate how you are enacting your beliefs and how you will continue to enact them. Two examples of integrative summaries follow (Exhibits 9.2 and 9.3):

---

**Exhibit 9.2**  Integrative Summary

I am comfortable with my teaching ability and am continuing to strive for educational excellence in the classroom and clinical areas. I have integrated the principles of emancipatory education into my teaching methodologies by increasing discussions and using case studies that foster critical thinking. I am enjoying the position that I have been granted at the hospital as co-chair of the Nursing Research Council and developing EBP projects with the staff. I use an emancipatory method to teach them about research and I have started a succession plan for that position by developing a 3-credit course that can be

*Continued*

**Exhibit 9.2**  *Continued*

taught by other faculty members to assist in keeping the program intact. My service to the department, university, and communities will continue. I will be instrumental on the undergraduate curriculum committee in its attempt to develop a new comprehensive nursing curriculum that includes the Institute of Medicine (IOM) goals and methodologies to increase critical thinking.

My research efforts will continue and I will focus on women's decision making as my key content area. Further studies to develop my theory of emancipated decision making will assist me to better understand the clinical realm of women's health, in which I teach and publish. I will attend further grant writing conferences to sharpen my grant-writing skills.

**Exhibit 9.3**  Integrative Summary

I have demonstrated excellence in teaching, professional scholarship, and service while in my position as instructor of nursing. I know I will bring to the position of Assistant Professor/tenure-track my passion for nursing and teaching, and I will continue my excellence in scholarship and service. I am committed to the future of nursing and Francis Marion University's priority of educational excellence to meet the needs of the Pee Dee Region and surrounding areas.

================*FAST FACTS in a NUTSHELL*

Continuing education steps that you have taken to increase success in areas that need improvement are also great to mention (Oermann, 2002).

## SELF-ASSESSMENT OF YOUR PORTFOLIO

Wilcox and Brown (2002) provide an evaluative mechanism for portfolios that provides an excellent self-assessment guide. The main points are as follows:

- Validity: Do your skills, accomplishments, and knowledge match the specifications of the job that you are in?
- Sufficiency: Is there enough evidence for the reviewers in order for them to make a judgment?
- Authentic: Is all of the work included clearly your own or have you misrepresented any portion of any project?
- Reliability: Will the evidence steer each evaluator to the same conclusions?
- Current: Is the evidence current and not anything you have done in the past and have not kept up?

Reflective questions that you should ask yourself are:

- What is the purpose of the portfolio?
- Who are the evaluators?
- What evidence would they expect?
- What evidence is most on target?
- What evidence will they weight the most?

## SUMMARY

The last part (*Part 5*) of your personal statement is the synthesis of your achievements and goals. It tells the evaluators what you are most proud of and what you will accomplish next. You should end your personal statement on a positive note that encourages your evaluators to share in your passion for your career.

═══════════════════════════════ *FAST FACTS in a NUTSHELL*

Ongoing outline of your academic portfolio:

1. Part 1: Preface/Abstract (approximately 1 page)
2. Part 2: Teaching (3–6 pages)
   a. Teaching Philosophy (1 of the 3–6 pages)
   b. Teaching Responsibilities
   c. Narrative About Teaching Scholarship
3. Part 3: Research and/or Scholarship (2–6 pages)
   a. Research Activities
   b. Publications and Presentations
4. Part 4: Service (2–3 pages)
   a. Departmental
   b. Institutional
   c. Community
5. Part 5: Integrative Summary (1–2 pages)
   a. Three Accomplishments
   b. Three Goals

# 10

## Arrangement and Presentation of Your Portfolio

### INTRODUCTION

*The method and design you use to organize and present your academic portfolio are very important. The best academic portfolios follow themes that stem from the nurse educators' teaching philosophies and use selective evidence to showcase the points or threads they would like highlighted (Murray, 1994).*

At the end of this chapter, the nurse educator will be able to:

1. Arrange the portfolio so that it is easily cross referenced.
2. Reflect on how each selective piece contributes to the telling of the professional journey.
3. Develop a table of contents.

## TABLE OF CONTENTS

Your portfolio should include a table of contents so that the reviewer knows what to expect and where to expect to find it (Melland & Volden, 1996; Morin, 2006). The table of contents also will assist you to evaluate the whole picture and to avoid developing an academic portfolio of excessive length (Melland & Volden, 1996). An example of a table of contents from my academic portfolio is provided in Exhibit 10.1.

**Exhibit 10.1    Table of Contents**

═══════════════════════*FAST FACTS in a NUTSHELL*

Melland and Volden (1996) recommend:

- Avoid using your portfolio as a dumping ground of artifacts.
- Balancing your artifacts or evidence with your personal statement.
- Avoid having many artifacts and too little to say and vice versa.

## USE OF HEADINGS AND FONTS

To guide the evaluators through each section of your personal statement, use the appropriate American

Psychological Association (APA) (APA, 2009) heading levels. This will help your thought process move smoothly from one part of your personal statement to the next.

It is also a good idea to follow APA formatting for font size and style. Double spacing is usually not necessary but will improve readability as will using extra space between sections. Margins that are the standard 1 inch work well, as does using a heavier weight paper.

## SUPPORT LETTERS

There are several types of support letters that can be included in an academic portfolio, including a letter from the department chairperson, unsolicited letters of support received by a faculty member, and letters of support from colleagues working in a clinical agency where you work.

- Each institution usually has a stipulation that the department chair must write a letter of support for promotion or tenure. That letter is usually weighted heavily in the evaluation process due to the fact the members of the evaluation committee are counting on the expertise of the department chair. Other faculty support letters may also be sought but should speak to knowing the performance of the candidate. Some evaluation teams also like to see support letters from faculty from other departments that attest to collaboration on university projects.
- Unsolicited letters also can be an important piece of evidence in an academic portfolio (Melland & Volden, 1999; Oermann, 1999). Support letters may be from students in progress or alumni and may be difficult to get if you have not collected them already.

There are ethical considerations governing the action of asking a student who has not graduated for a support letter. Clinical agency personnel are another source of support letters and can attest to your teaching in the clinical area. Most nurses have professional relationships with managers, administrators, and staff nurses on the nursing care units where they teach. Choose a few letters that speak directly to the skills you are highlighting in your personal statement.

## PRESENTATION OF YOUR PORTFOLIO

An academic portfolio, regardless of the container you choose to use (i.e., binder, folder, or file box), needs to look professional and have dividers to organize the personal statement, curriculum vitae, and each section of the appendices: teaching, research or scholarship, and service. A three-ring binder with pockets keeps your portfolio organized and delivers your portfolio in a professional manner. It is best to use one container or binder for your portfolio, because your portfolio will be passed around during the evaluation process. A binder will decrease the chance that pieces will become separated.

### *FAST FACTS in a NUTSHELL*

Remember to make your academic portfolio as professional looking as possible—it is not a scrapbooking project!

Once you have completed your portfolio, it is a good idea to ask a mentor, several colleagues, or peers to review it critically before you formally submit it to the administration or the human resource department.

================================*FAST FACTS in a NUTSHELL*

Most important—have a mentor look at your portfolio (Oermann, 1999).

## SUMMARY

This chapter provided nurse educators with clues about the
professional presentation of their portfolio. Understanding
that appearance is important when striving for advancement is the theoretical underpinnings of this emphasis.
Many nurse educators are very creative but creativity
should be limited in the development of this product. The
next chapter is contributed and will discuss the development of e-portfolios, as some institutions are requesting
academic portfolios in electronic format versus the traditional type. Chapters 12 and 13 present excellent examples of personal statements from nurse educators. The
example presented in Chapter 12 was used successfully
to gain promotion from instructor to assistant professor
rank in a state-funded liberal arts college. The example
in Chapter 13 was used successfully to secure tenure in
a research intensive institution. The Appendix provides
biographical data on the contributors of this book to give
some insight into their career tracks and aspirations.

# How to Develop an e-Portfolio

Dr. Frances H. Cornelius

## INTRODUCTION

*Electronic portfolios (e-portfolios) have evolved to become much more than creatively presented resumes or scrapbooks (e-Portfolios, 2002) and can "facilitate the transition between institutions and stages of education," as well as "supporting staff appraisal and applications for professional accreditation" (Joint Information Systems Committee, 2008, p. 5). e-Portfolios have the capability to show reflection, evolution of thought, and professional development in a very engaging and often interactive interface. The concurrent explosive growth of the World Wide Web (www) and its transformative effect upon how we find and consume information has also had an impact upon the growing acceptance of the e-portfolio. Kimball (2003) states that the very qualities that have contributed to the success of the web—"its graphical nature and ability to support links between digital artifacts"—make it a perfect medium to present a professional portfolio. Whether you use these capabilities to publish your*

> *portfolio on the web or you keep it on a local hard drive, CD, or thumb drive, the outcome is the same. These technologies provide an effective way to present yourself in the* best possible light *while requiring only the very basic technical savvy.*

At the end of this chapter the nurse educator will be able to:

1. Discuss differences between traditional hard-copy portfolios and e-portfolios.
2. Describe alternatives for e-portfolios and criteria to aid the selection process.
3. Understand how to get started setting up an e-portfolio.

## OVERVIEW

e-Portfolios have been widely used in education, particularly in K–12, to assess student performance as well as document teaching competencies. The format provides a very effective means for presenting teaching/learning experiences and competencies. For example, consider the following scenario described on the Advanced Learning Technologies–Center for Research on Learning at the University of Kansas website:

When the newly minted teacher sat down for a job interview in her school district, she flipped open her laptop computer and began her presentation. Here, she said, was a statement of her teaching philosophy—and an iMovie clip of her applying that philosophy to a lesson plan. Click. Here was a description of a state teaching and technology standard—and a hotlink to a website that her students developed as a class project. Click. And here too was a diary entry, telling of her student residency in a rural village, and a letter she'd sent non-English-speaking parents, asking them to join a classroom celebration of multicultural diversity.

The wrap-around effect was effective. So effective, in fact, that the school principal hired her on the spot. (e-Portfolios, 2002, ¶ 1–2)

## BENEFITS OF E-PORTFOLIOS

Clearly, e-portfolios offer considerable advantages over the traditional "hard copy" portfolios. The e-portfolio can provide a very engaging method of highlighting your accomplishments, teaching philosophy, and capabilities, thereby maximizing your opportunities for career advancement whether the goal is a new position or a promotion. This format can provide a user-friendly entry point that can effectively welcome and guide your reviewer through your portfolio (Figure 11.1).

The main advantage of an e-portfolio is that it is digital and therefore can be easily modified and updated in

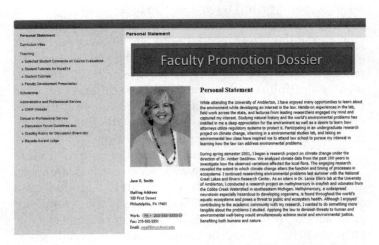

**FIGURE 11.1** Sample Faculty Promotion e-Portfolio.

contrast with the more static, traditional, hard-copy portfolio. This dynamic characteristic also allows you to more easily make changes to tailor your portfolio for a particular prospective employer and to demonstrate and/or update competencies in various areas.

An e-portfolio will contain the usual content typically found in the hard copy teaching portfolio, as described in Chapter 2, including: (1) curriculum vitae (CV), (2) teaching philosophy, (3) career plan, (4) grants (submitted or awarded), (5) teaching examples (PowerPoint presentation or other representative teaching materials), and (6) sample writings and publication, and can be organized as described in Chapter 8. While traditional portfolios focus on the presentation of written work, the e-portfolio can include multimedia—graphics, audio, and video—providing more options for showcasing what you have accomplished.

The real power in the digital format is that you are not restricted in how the content is organized—you can arrange your materials in any manner that "fits" the objective of the particular presentation. As mentioned, you can tailor your portfolio to emphasize particular aspects/accomplishments that highlight you as the best possible candidate for a specific position or appointment. e-Portfolios make it easier to have different types of portfolios—for example, you can have a one that focuses on your "best work" and another that highlights your professional growth and development over time.

In addition, the digital format allows content to be more easily organized or re-organized, more easily searchable, and *highly transportable*—you can carry it around on a thumb drive, burn it to a CD, or store it the "cloud" for easy access from any location that has internet access. Other benefits include the ability to store materials safely and securely, in pristine condition—no more searching for missing materials!

Also, with very little effort, new items can easily replace older work. As Billings and Kowalski (2008) maintain, keeping the portfolio up-to-date is essential, no matter what format you use. "The portfolio should be updated regularly.... If the portfolio is not updated regularly, it can be time consuming to do after the fact.... Key information may be lost or forgotten and not readily available when requested on short notice" (p. 533). The true value of the digital format is that these "tweaks" can be easily accomplished, particularly if you do as Billings recommends and set a regular appointment reminder on your calendar.

Another clear benefit is that when you present yourself using an e-portfolio, you are demonstrating that you have computer and technical skills. These skills are highly valued by employers and are frequently viewed as essential competencies for a technology infused workplace.

## LEVERAGING THE POWER OF WWW TOOLS

Because e-portfolios are stored digitally, the content takes up very little physical space while still containing a great deal of information. When you have a lot of information, it is absolutely essential to organize and connect components in a meaningful way. In an e-portfolio, components can be interconnected via hyperlinks, making it easier to provide supplemental information to support statements you make within the portfolio and for the reviewer to make important connections with the content. This allows you to explain the *context* of the artifacts. Presenting artifacts in isolation does not effectively convey to your reviewer the significance or relevance of the items, or how each relates to and builds upon the other. For example, consider the presentation of content in Figure 11.2. In this area, the faculty member utilized hyperlinks to provide supportive documentation and further explanation of concepts

A competency based curriculum requires a mix of didactic and experiential learning activities, all of which must actively engage the learner. I develop assignments to challenge students at each level of Bloom's Taxonomy of cognitive levels.

Below are some examples of assignments that demonstrate:

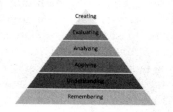

- Creating - Group I <u>Final Project</u>
- Evaluating - <u>Website Evaluation</u>
- Analyzing - Douglass High <u>Reaction Paper</u>
- Applying - <u>Case Study</u>- Recovery & Relapse Prev.
- Understanding - <u>What's in your suitcase</u>?
- Remembering - <u>Exam 1</u> for psychopharm

Another helpful teaching formula is "<u>ROPES</u>". This is effective in situations where students have no clinical experience with a particular topic. "ROPES" helps the students connect their everyday experiences to the topic and insures that unfamiliar terms, and concepts are adequately explained.

This <u>PowerPoint</u> presentation from Class #1 of Child Psychopathology is a good example of how I use the Review and Overview method to engage students in the course material.

This next PowerPoint presentation from BACS 405 Family Focused Interventions is an <u>example</u> of the presentation and exercise phase of a lesson. Students learn about the ABCX model of family adaptation and then they talk with a family about their strengths, beliefs, resources and coping strategies. In class, we review the homework exercise, connecting their expereince back to the concepts of the model.

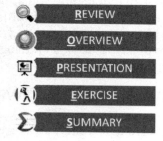

The Psychiatric Rehabilitation Practitioner must be an expert at teaching skills. Many people who need psychiatric rehabilitation services have cognitive impairments that present barriers to learning. Thus, one simple approach to teaching skills is the tell-show-do method. Here is an <u>example of a curriculum</u> I developed to teach staff of CareLink how to teach skills using the tell-show-do method.

I use this method to help students master skills as well. Here is an <u>example</u> of the tell-show-do method applied to a learning module on psychiatric rehabilitation diagnosing. The PowerPoint is the "tell" step, the case example is the "show" step and the mini-project assignment is the "do" step.

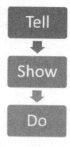

# FIGURE 11.2    Sample Presentation of Teaching Including Hyperlinks and Images.

Reprinted with permission of Lisa Schmidt, PhD, MA, BA.

referred to in the body of the text. This technique, as well as the use of images, provides a user interface that is impossible to replicate in the traditional hard copy format. It is the ability to *make connections between the artifacts* that is the true power of the e-portfolio. Hyperlinking between artifacts provides an effective mechanism to make meaningful connections between your education, teaching, scholarship, and service experience. These connections can be supported through reflective statements and brief explanations that make it clear to the reviewer how the artifacts relate to each other as examples of your accomplishments, skills, competencies, and professional growth and development. The key objective is, of course, showcasing your best work and documenting your growth and development over time.

## E-PORTFOLIOS

There are three approaches that can be utilized when creating an e-portfolio. These include using (1) a proprietary e-portfolio product, ( 2) a personal learning environment (PLE), or (3) a Web page editor (or HTML editor).

The first option is the easiest way to create an e-portfolio. Using a product that has been specifically designed for the purpose allows you to get up and running very quickly by using imbedded templates and tools. There are a variety of e-portfolios available on the market today. Often, these are provided at a nominal fee for individual users; there are also a few that offer free or free limited accounts with the option to upgrade to a "for fee" product. For a sampling of currently available e-portfolio products, please refer to Table 11.1.

**TABLE 11.1** Examples of Available e-Portfolio Products

| Product Name | Developer | Web Address | Cost |
| --- | --- | --- | --- |
| Digi[cation] | Digication | http://www.digication.com | Free |
| eFolioWorld | Avenet eFolio | http://www.efolioworld.com | Fee based |
| Epsilen | Epsilen LLC | http://www.epsilen.com | Free for education professionals |
| ePortfolio.org | ePortfolio.org | http://www.eportfolio.org | Fee based |
| FolioSpaces | FolioSpaces | http://www.foliospaces.com | Free; upgrade available |
| Interfolio | Interfolio, Inc. | http://www.interfolio.com | Fee based |
| iWebfolio | Nuventive | http://www.nuventive.com | Fee based |
| Rcampus | Reazons Systems, Inc. | http://www.rcampus.com | Free |

================*FAST FACTS in a NUTSHELL*

Some of the clear benefits of using an e-portfolio product include:

- Quick start templates
- Capability to create multiple e-portfolios for different purposes
- Easy integration of multimedia and links
- Controlled reviewer and guest access, with capability to selectively issue invitations
- Quick post and update capabilities
- Secure, centralized storage of artifacts

The second option still utilizes available imbedded tools but involves re-purposing a web environment for the purpose. A PLE is defined by Lubensky (December 2006) as a **"facility for an individual to access, aggregate, configure and manipulate digital artifacts of their ongoing learning experiences"** (¶ 5). PLEs, such as Netvibes (http://www.netvibes.com) or Pageflakes (http://www.pageflakes.com), are free, web-based environments that provide resources/tools to manage, organize, and present materials.

The third option available to those of you who are slightly more adventurous and technically savvy, is to use freely available tools that allow you to create an e-portfolio. What you would need to get started is a web page editor (Table 11.2). Web page editors are actually imbedded within the e-portfolio products and the PLEs listed above, but if you want to create your own portfolio, you will need at a minimum a web page (HTML) editor. HTML editors have built-in WYSIWYG functionality, which stands for "what you see is what you get." This means that you do not need to know HTML to write or edit your pages. These editors function similarly to a typical word processing

**TABLE 11.2** Sampling of Free HTML Editors

| HTML Editor | URL | Operating System |
|---|---|---|
| Alleycode | http://www.alleycode.com | Windows |
| Amaya | http://www.w3.org/Amaya | Windows, MacOS, Unix |
| Aptana Studio | http://www.aptana.org/products/studio2 | MacOS |
| Bluefish | http://bluefish.openoffice.nl | Windows, Linux, FreeBSD, MacOS-X, OpenBSD, Solaris |
| Komodo Edit | http://www.activestate.com/komodo-edit | MacOS |
| KompoZer | http://kompozer.net | Windows, MacOS-X, GNU/Linux |
| NetBeans IDE | http://netbeans.org | Windows, Linux, MacOS-X and Solaris |
| SeaMonkey | http://www.seamonkey-project.org | Windows, MacOS |

program such as Microsoft Word, so they are very easy to use. All you need is some basic word processing skills and to start typing!

## GETTING STARTED WITH AN E-PORTFOLIO

As with a traditional portfolio, the first step is to gather all relevant materials except for an e-portfolio, you will need to get your materials in a digital format. If you have documents, such as certificates, awards or publications, in hard copy, you will need to scan these. All the materials you collect, whether word documents, PDFs, images, video files, podcasts, or other multimedia content, can be collectively referred to as *artifacts*. These artifacts should be stored in one place so that you easily locate and manage your materials, as well as see your professional growth and development over time. It is important to note that if you decide to use an established e-portfolio product, you may be required to upload your artifacts to a "library," which will store your materials securely and also allow you to easily select various artifacts to place within your portfolio.

*FAST FACTS in a NUTSHELL*

Select your artifacts carefully:

- What was the context of the artifact? What does it represent/highlight?
- What/when was this artifact created? For what purpose?
- What does the artifact mean to you? Why is it important to include in your portfolio?
- What does this artifact show about you? How does it highlight your capabilities?

Once you have all the artifacts collected and centrally located, you are ready to get started working on your portfolio. At this point, it is helpful to have some kind of organizational structure mocked-up to help with the design and appropriate placement of your materials. First make a list of the materials you have collected and develop an outline.

An important next step in this process is to consider who your audience may be and anticipate how best to present your materials. Will the portfolio be used to secure a new position at a new college or university? In this case, you may wish to highlight those accomplishments that more closely match the information on the job posting and the college or university's mission statement. Or, if the audience would be reviewing your portfolio for promotion/tenure, you can organize your portfolio to match the criteria for promotion. Remember, if your audience changes, you can easily modify the portfolio to meet the need—that is the beauty of it!

## *FAST FACTS in a NUTSHELL*

To get started putting together your e-portfolio:

- Make a list of your artifacts (materials you have collected).
- Organize your list using an outline.
- Consider the type of portfolio you are creating (showcase vs. professional growth and development).
- Rank your artifacts based upon the criteria established by the type of portfolio you are creating and assemble them for optimal presentation.
- Review criteria and make a list of additional artifacts or revisions needed.

## SUMMARY

The use of portfolios in nursing is gaining momentum and is viewed as a strategy to not only support continuing education, but also as a method to collect and present evidence of professional growth and development. e-Portfolios are becoming more widely used and are considered by many to be an integral technology to support life-long learning (Norman & George, 2006). It is clear that e-portfolios are here to stay and should be embraced as a tremendous opportunity for you to manage your career.

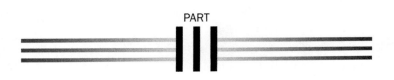

PART

III

# Examples

# 12

## Personal Statement for Promotion From Instructor to Assistant Professor

### Dr. Karen K. Gittings

## INTRODUCTION

*The candidate or personal statement is an extremely important part of the portfolio for promotion. Because this statement is located in the beginning of the portfolio, it is usually the first document to be read by evaluators. This statement should provide an overview of the candidate's accomplishments in the areas of teaching, scholarship, and service. It serves to showcase the candidate and identify why the candidate is deserving of promotion.*

*Getting started with the personal statement is often the hardest part. It is helpful to divide records into separate files for teaching, scholarship, and service. Important accomplishments should be selected from each category for inclusion in the personal statement. Depending upon the mission of the parent institution, it may be appropriate to focus more heavily in one area than another.*

*Many nurse educators will find it difficult to write a personal statement of their accomplishments. The statement needs to be written in a bold, positive fashion that highlights accomplishments and minimizes areas needing improvement. Candidates may view this statement as embellishing or bragging, but self-promotion is vital in helping the evaluators learn about the candidate and make decisions for promotion. A bold, strong personal statement of accomplishments will greatly improve chances of promotion.*

At the end of this chapter, the nurse educator will be able to:

1. Appraise a personal statement used for promotion.
2. Extract presentation points that would enhance their own academic portfolio.
3. Develop a sense of how an academic portfolio should read to a reviewer.

The following illustrates a Personal Statement for Promotion.

## Karen K. Gittings

## CANDIDATE STATEMENT

I am currently seeking promotion from Nursing Instructor to Assistant Professor in the Department of Nursing at Francis Marion University. After working for one semester as an adjunct clinical instructor and completing my Master's of Science in Nursing (MSN) degree with a major in Nursing Education in the fall of 2006, I was hired as a full-time nursing instructor in January of 2007. At the completion of the fall 2010 semester, I will have completed 4 years of full-time service to Francis Marion University. During these 4 years of service, I have learned, grown, and developed in my faculty role. I have met all the criteria for Assistant Professor, and I respectfully request that I be considered for promotion.

### Preface Critique

*In her preface, Dr. Gittings gives a brief history to bring reviewers up-to-date on where she has been. She is positive about what the educational institution has provided her and, most importantly, she is very clear about the objective for submitting her academic portfolio.*

## Teaching

My teaching knowledge and skills are a personal strong point. The primary course in which I coordinate and have teaching responsibilities is NURS 407: Adult Health II. In this course, I teach 3 hours per week in the classroom and 9 hours per week in the clinical setting at Carolinas Hospital System. Because my clinical expertise is critical care and care of cardiac patients, I also guest lecture every semester on cardiac related topics in NURS 406: Synthesis and NURS 305: Pharmacology. Last semester, I co-coordinated and had primary teaching responsibilities in NURS 310: Adult Health I. I have also taught in the clinical setting for NURS 304: Fundamentals and Adult Health I, NURS 406: Synthesis, and was a guest lecturer and taught a lab in NURS 301: Health Assessment. I am also a member of the Department of Nursing Simulation Team, and I have been teaching IV simulation with senior level nursing students, and I demonstrated teaching of IV simulation to two MUSC graduate level nursing students.

Students in my course have been required to complete community service hours with agencies that serve the vulnerable, uninsured, and/or underserved in the Pee Dee region. Through self-reflection and journaling, students are encouraged to further develop their caring behaviors. Students are also taught the importance of giving back to their community and those in need. Through this community service program, I have been able to develop solid working relationships with community agencies such as the Free Medical Clinic of Darlington County, Harvest Hope Food Bank, Hope Health, and Pee Dee Coalition.

Students have provided positive feedback on course and clinical evaluations. My student evaluations are consistently excellent-to-good. I have been honored to be asked to introduce three students at their Phi Kappa Phi inductions. Perhaps my greatest honor, though, was being awarded the "Outstanding Clinical Caring Teacher Award" by the May 2009 graduating class (Department of Nursing) and the "Outstanding Faculty Caring Teacher Award" by the December 2010 graduating class (Department of Nursing).

My level of teaching expertise has continually been increased by my attending many nursing related conferences that serve to strengthen my clinical knowledge, as well as keep my nursing knowledge current and relevant for teaching in the classroom setting. Since 1991, I have continuously held my certification in critical care nursing (CCRN), which requires validation of knowledge every 3 years. More recently, I have started attending education-related conferences, seminars, and webinars that cover information on pedagogical skill, teaching techniques, curriculum design, and evaluation.

## Teaching Critique

Dr. Gittings describes what she does and how she does in her role as a faculty member. She is space limited by her educational institution so there was not so much an

emphasis on philosophy as there was on her accomplishments. She has also integrated aspects of service into the
discussion of guest lecturing. As previously stated, there
are overlapping areas in any academic portfolio. One
excellent point that Dr. Gittings makes in this section is
her commitment to learning how to increase her skill as
a nurse educator. This demonstrates her accountability to
her position and she can add a select example of the conference brochures to place in the appendix to support her
statements.

## Scholarship

In May 2010, I graduated from Duquesne University with
a Doctor in Nursing Practice (DNP) degree with a focus
in Nursing Education; my GPA upon graduation was a
4.0. During my doctoral program, I was inducted into Phi
Kappa Phi at Duquesne University. I also retain membership in Sigma Theta Tau International, Honor Society of
Nursing.

I presented my capstone project, *"Developing Caring
Behaviors in Undergraduate, Baccalaureate Nursing Students
Through Planned Community Service Experiences,"* in May
of 2010 to peers, the faculty of the School of Nursing at
Duquesne University, and invited guests. I have also dis-
cussed organ donation with the general public as part of
an informational booth at "She Saturday" in Florence.
I am also a co-presenter for a session on "Intravenous
Education Through Simulation" at Drexel University's
*Simulation in Healthcare: Where No One Has Gone Before*
conference on March 25, 2011, in Orlando, Florida.

As part of the Department of Nursing's self-study for
reaccreditation, I am the team leader and co-author for
Standard 2 (Faculty and Staff). Currently, I am actively
involved in the nursing department's Publication Club,

and I have peer-reviewed faculty articles for journal submission. I am also the second author for an article titled "Nurses' Perceptions of How Their Body Art is Interpreted," which has been accepted for publication in *Nursing2010*.

### Scholarship Critique

*Dr. Gittings's scholarship section shows growth. It began with her educational journey, which can be assumed to have taken up most of her time. But after she completed her doctorate, she began publishing and presenting. That transition from student to scholar without a long lapse in time says mountains about her commitment and motivation!*

## Service

My service to Francis Marion University, the Department of Nursing, the profession of nursing, and my community has been multifaceted. I have conducted several open houses at Francis Marion University and spoke to potential students and parents about the nursing program. In the clinical setting, I constantly remind my students that we represent Francis Marion University, and I often speak to patients, families, and hospital staff about the university and nursing program, and have recruited RN-to-BSN students.

In the Department of Nursing, I participate in many committees. Since August 2009, I have been the Chair of the Evaluation and Program Improvement (EPI) Committee; in this role, I had a significant part in the research, purchase, and launch of our alumni and employer surveys. I report to the Nursing Advisory Committee related to EPI issues. Other committees of which I am currently a member include the Faculty Committee, NLNAC Committee, and Medical-Surgical Committee. I previously served on the KATTS (Knowledge Base, Anxiety Control, Test-Taking Skills) Committee and Curriculum Threads and Outcomes Sub-Committee. I have attended the last three Palmetto Gold Banquets to support our nursing students who were receiving an awarded scholarship.

I have served my profession by remaining involved in the American Association of Critical-Care Nurses (AACN). I attend local meetings of the Pee Dee Area Chapter of AACN, and I served as President-Elect from 2006–2007 and President from 2007–2008. I was recently elected to a 2-year term as Vice President of the Francis Marion University Department of Nursing Honor Society.

To serve my community, I volunteer monthly at the Free Medical Clinic of Darlington County. In this role, I triage clients, provide education, and counsel about other community resources. I also try to work at least 12 hours a month in the Cardiovascular Intensive Care Unit (CVICU) at Carolinas Hospital System to retain my critical care nursing skills.

### Service Critique

*Dr. Gittings's service statement is excellent in the areas of departmental and community service. She discusses how she assists the department, as well as how she assists the community in health-related activities. It shows commitment to the profession that is enhanced by university service, which is sometimes difficult to acquire. To be voted onto a university committee to lend service is a process that takes time, socialization with the rest of the academic community members, and for some committees—tenure.*

## Summary

To summarize, in the 4 years that I have been at Francis Marion University, I have a proven record of teaching excellence, scholarship, and service. I am proud to represent Francis Marion University, and I truly enjoy all aspects of my faculty role in the Department of Nursing. Thank you for considering my request for promotion to Assistant Professor.

---

## SUMMARY

This chapter presented a bold, positive personal statement along with critiques of each major section. Although nurse educators may be reluctant initially to showcase their accomplishments, it is vital in attaining promotion. The personal statement led to the successful promotion of the author from Nursing Instructor to Assistant Professor of Nursing.

# 13

## Personal Statement for Continuous Tenure

### Dr. Roberta Waite

## INTRODUCTION

*Personal statements for tenure are a powerful tool to showcase one's strengths and the arduous work applicants have invested over the course of a typical period of 6 years. Your personal statement is a critical reflection of three central areas—teaching, research and scholarship, and service. An understanding of your academic institution's philosophy and mission is critical when sculpting your statement. That is, most research intensive or very high research intensive schools require substantial evidence of success and rigor in scholarship and research, while performance in the areas of teaching and service need to be at least satisfactory.*

At the end of this chapter, the nurse educator will be able to:

1. Understand the writing style needed for academic portfolios.
2. Discuss the components of an extensive personal statement.
3. Identify themes throughout the portfolio and how they are integrated in the last section.

Evasive and passive language should be avoided when framing your work and describing your professional image and research trajectory. Deliberate inclusion of valid information is important, such as (1) noting how your contributions align with advancing the mission of the school; (2) indicating innovative strategies that you have developed; and (3) highlighting how the programmatic nature of your research has had an impact locally, regionally, nationally, and/or globally. Also, emphasis on the collaborative nature of work can be invaluable. This is a document where you want to accentuate your positive qualities.

There are several additional factors that need to be considered when developing your personal statement. Always review the university's tenure guidelines and examine portfolios of recently tenured faculty. University guidelines tend to be vague; however, you want to ensure you have a framework upon which to build your statement. Recently tenured faculty also set the standard and therefore serve as a benchmark for what is expected particularly in your department. Understanding this is paramount because how one interprets excellence may vary. Be sure to compare your statement with someone of similar position (i.e., not a person seeking tenure who primarily had an administrative position). While excelling in the central three target areas is requisite, remember that the personal statement and tenure process are political. Standards for tenure at institutions often shift and individual interpretations among peers on the tenure committee can vary, particularly as some of these committees may be interdisciplinary.

Lastly, whenever possible have documented data about any information cited in your personal statement.

Granting tenure is a major undertaking by any academic institution. Therefore, once you have obtained the appropriate success in the aforementioned areas, write your personal statement in a manner that will negate any question about awarding you tenure on the part of the internal and external review committees and the administration. The following section illustrates how I documented my personal statement when I applied for tenure and promotion to associate professor within a research intensive university.

## Roberta Waite, EdD, APRN, CNS-BC

## PERSONAL STATEMENT FOR PROMOTION AND TENURE

In this personal statement I will present the evolution of my professional development while in pursuit of a tenured and associate professor position at Drexel University. This has been my first academic position. Needless to say this position has offered significant challenges and opportunities given that I had not (1) previously taught in a class setting (online or in person) other than providing in-service training, (2) conducted research other than my doctoral dissertation, (3) submitted any publications, and (4) presented at any peer-reviewed professional presentations. I was recruited to Drexel University, College of Nursing and Health Professions (CNHP), as a full-time (12 months per year) faculty member in 2003 after having worked in an urban clinical setting as a clinician and administrator for 15 years. Initially recruited for a faculty position to work in the undergraduate nursing program that was flourishing from an increased enrollment of over 800 students, I taught student populations in the 5-year Co-Operative, 11-month Accelerated Career Entry (ACE), and online Registered Nurse-Bachelors of Science in Nursing (RN-BSN) Programs. The nursing programs now have over 1,800 students and have expanded to include a Doctor of Nursing Practice program. In 2007, I started teaching in the master's and doctoral nursing programs. It has been an honor and remarkable opportunity to relate my nursing experiences to students in the classroom, at clinical sites, and online, by teaching a variety of courses in the undergraduate and now graduate nursing programs. During the past 6 years, I have had the opportunity to (1) develop and challenge my teaching skills, (2) increase my scholarship and research productivity, and (3) expand upon my service activities within the nursing profession and academic community. The development of my research has expanded to include a public/community mental health focus. As such, I was invited by Dr. Gerrity, the Director of the Eleventh Street Family Health Services Center, to take a research scientist position at the Center in July of 2008. I also serve as associate faculty in the Center for Health Equality, School of Public Health at Drexel University. My work at the University supports my professional goals of enhancing student involvement in scholarship and research, teaching at varied levels and across disciplines, and engaging students in both applying cultural competence to practice and research. This is critical given the diverse communities and vulnerable populations served in health care and community settings. I am pleased to have the opportunity to present an overview of my accomplishments in teaching, research and scholarship, and service, and to share my future plans.

## Preface Critique

*Dr. Waite does a similar exercise as in the previously critiqued preface. She "lays it out" for the reviewers. She effectively describes where she is coming from and where she is headed professionally. She tells them exactly why she is presenting her portfolio and entices the reviewers to want to read more by indicating that her future plans will be revealed.*

## TEACHING

### Teaching Overview

I came into teaching from the role of a nurse clinician and administrator. Having experienced over 15 years in these roles, I am acutely aware of the significant contribution registered nurses can make in changing the life conditions, interpersonal experiences, and behavioral characteristics that create struggles for individuals, families, and communities. My intention in teaching future and current registered nurses is to ensure they are equipped with the values, knowledge, and skills to make certain that their contribution in a helping relationship with clients is a positive one. Given that I teach across multiple educational levels (DrNP, Masters in Nursing, and undergraduate for both licensed and unlicensed students), and both in-person and online courses, these principles shape my engagement with students at all stages. Currently my primary appointment is in the doctoral nursing program; however, I continue to teach undergraduate and master's level nursing students.

When I enter a classroom at the beginning of the quarter the weight is on me to establish that our purpose is to be, for however brief a time, a community of learners together. It positions me as a learner. But I am also not suggesting that I don't have more power. And I'm not trying to say we're all equal here. I'm trying to say that we are all equal here to the extent that we are equally committed to creating a learning environment.

bell hooks

## Teaching Philosophy and Methodologies

My belief is that teaching is a process, an evolving activity that spreads wisdom, imparts professional knowledge, and promotes academic excellence. The journey and craft of teaching requires competency and effectiveness that stem from reflection, commitment, passion, subject knowledge, experience, and, above all, a focus on students and their learning. Fundamentally, I have a progressive view of education and three threads of thought shape my philosophy of teaching: (1) *connection* with students, (2) *sharing* knowledge and responsibility for learning, and (3) *action and reflection*. These threads interplay through my commitment to critical thinking and integration of theory and practice. They also shape interactions with students when relating teaching and research concepts and reflection and development activities. My approach to teaching actualizes this philosophy through the use of interactive and experiential techniques in the classroom and through online synchronous and asynchronous learning environments. Each of these threads will be discussed briefly.

## Connection With Students

Through my commitment to know, connect with students, and guide their learning process, I create an environment where learning is facilitated in a safe environment. To facilitate contact and close the distance between students and faculty, I like to understand the individual student. This entails understanding the student's learning styles, background, and prior knowledge in the subject. To achieve this degree of individual understanding, I strive for a high level of interaction with my students in an atmosphere of friendly cooperation. Connecting with students beyond focusing on grades alone is important. This is a continual challenge; however, this investment demonstrates respect for individuals as humans and often helps relate respect for high expectations, which they can expect from me and me from them. One of my most valuable roles as an educator lies in my ability and willingness to connect with students to facilitate their learning. That means building connections to help students problematize the issues beyond the immediate parameters of their personal experiences and to help them understand that there are never any easy answers—I support them to question and rework many of their own assumptions. Students have to be encouraged to move beyond themselves to make the wider connections. I have to help them, therefore, develop informed perspectives that take into account multiple points of view but are also coherent and defensible.

Regarding online courses, connectivity is enhanced with telephone calls to students generally at least once per quarter in addition to routine asynchronous and synchronous sessions. Students often comment on evaluations, "Dr. Waite is very approachable and really makes sure you understand everything. I really like how she personally called me at the beginning of the semester to make sure I understood all the material." For online classes, I also have students participate in a class photo-op and arrange for a student café in Blackboard for students to dialogue outside of scheduled class time. The class photo-op enables students to "see" who their colleagues are as they engage throughout the quarter, and the café helps students build relationships with colleagues. Taking the time to implement these strategies has been crucial to building a community given the lack of human in-person contact with students and for students to be able to dialogue and share with each other as they might in a traditional class setting.

## Sharing Knowledge and Responsibility for Learning

In my experience, I find that too often many students would rather be told what to do, accomplish the task, receive a grade, and leave. Given my educational philosophy, I value students who see the greater possibilities of knowledge. I want them to consider the content presented to them for what counts as knowledge and how we justify what we name as knowledge through critical discussion. Underlying my teaching philosophy is the belief that it is more important to have students learn *how* to think than *what* to think. Individuals with theoretical frameworks, infinite wisdom, and core influences that have helped to shape and challenge my own philosophy include Paulo Freire, Kurt Hahn, bell hooks, and John Dewey. Freire emphasized social justice and education for liberation of the oppressed; he also preached that any constructive dialogue involves (and demands) respect. Hahn believed education calls for the deepest qualities of character and compassion. The work of bell hooks helps guide teaching practices in a multicultural environment and creates a space where students of all backgrounds can become independent thinkers in the arena of a dominant European culture of decision makers. Dewey's ability to weave his moral compass into science and the art of education captures me. Utilizing these philosophical viewpoints and connecting with students as people are critical given that knowledge itself cannot be transmitted in the same form from teacher to student, but rather, knowledge is constructed by the student in a complex integration of prior experience, existing knowledge, and new experience.

Knowledge is power that helps shape who we are and empowers us to enhance our unique sense of self and community. Therefore, I have endeavored to push students to think critically, self-examine, take risks for learning purposes, and challenge the validity of all knowledge being presented to make certain they are both consumers and creators of knowledge. Students should be engaged with alternative viewpoints that challenge existing assumptions and encourage critical thinking. I find it exciting when students are able to move beyond parroting what the textbook or I tell them and are able to draw their own conclusions from the material. I encourage students to learn how to apply knowledge within a cultural context and emphasize the significance of cultural competence in today's nursing practice world. While holding students to high standards, I also endeavor to create a safe, nurturing, learning environment that provides permission for students to share their knowledge (or lack thereof), their struggles, their triumphs, and their fears about the topic being discussed or their practice with clients in the respective settings. I hold students to high standards in their behavior and deportment in the classroom (in-person or online), their attention to assignments, and the quality of their work. The process of learning has become even more dynamic, as geographical area and/or domain is no longer limiting because of online learning. I believe this requires students to become more self-motivated and functionally literate. When I design the learning space and course content, I look for proactive strategies to make what I am teaching personal, relevant, and meaningful to the students. This occurs by sharing professional stories, using examples (e.g., current nursing events, policies, guest speakers), and integrating activities that relate to where students are in their program and life state, and by asking students to draw from their own experiences to situate learning and enrich classroom discussion. Setting the stage for engagement, connectivity, developing a community of learners, and engaging in open and critical discourse is essential. This approach is congruous with the mission of Drexel University (Drexel, 2011): "Students need to be engaged in education that is rigorous, relevant and learner-friendly."

Additional learner-oriented strategies that I utilize when teaching (e.g., small group activities, student-identified topics for papers, scholarly dialogue, collaborative student investigations, lecture, discussion, collaborative learning activities facilitated with the use of various technologies and instructional aids— film clips, PowerPoint, concept mapping, vignettes, case studies, one-minute papers, and team debates) promote development of knowledge that is both purposeful and enduring. These approaches support mutual knowledge sharing where a reciprocal relationship for learning process naturally evolves between me and the students in any particular course. This type of relationship is one that I cultivate not only between myself and the students, but also among the students themselves as I impress upon them that they, themselves, are also sources for knowledge and thus have the capacity for life-long learning—a necessity for skilled, responsible practitioners, good nurse clinicians, and researchers. Through the study of nursing, I seek to empower students to be better citizens and to provide them with the skills necessary to play a positive and educated role in society.

## Reflection and Action

As an educator, teaching, which itself is a learning activity, also involves focused reflection. My philosophy is that reflective skills are important skills for nursing students to acquire and for faculty to embrace and develop. Reflective practice helps both groups to understand other people's experiences and to facilitate helping relationships. Moreover, the development of the self is the foundation of becoming a professional. Reflection can be seen as a way to take a step back and think about a situation and one's self to gain a new perspective on a situation. With reflective thinking, students can construct meaning and knowledge that guide their actions in practice. In addition, reflection is a way of overcoming the divergence between theory and practice and a strategy to develop knowledge embedded within practice. Specific strategies used with students include reflective papers and journals, one-minute papers using reflection to draw meaning from clinical experience, and dialogue to help identify clinical and learning priorities. I believe that one cannot know what one knows until one has the opportunity to reflect upon one's experiences. When appropriate, I use my personal and clinical experiences to help students reflect and act in order to grasp information, make connections between extant literature and real life, and also to challenge my students to reflect on their thoughts and behaviors. Students have often expressed during classroom discussions that it was through these reflection opportunities that they came to synthesize and integrate their new skills and knowledge, enabling application of these skills across assignments, projects, discourses, and courses.

## Teaching Responsibilities

I have taught 10 different courses over the past 6 years. Four courses were for non-licensed undergraduate nursing students, three courses were in the RN to BSN program, one course was in the master's of education program, and two were doctoral nursing courses. In accordance with my midpoint review, teaching within the graduate program was a goal. I have chaired a graduate master's course (N599), 2006–2009, and this year the director of the doctoral nursing program appointed me track coordinator and course chair of a doctoral course (N835). I have enjoyed teaching in all programs and have received strong student evaluations as indicated in my yearly evaluations and midpoint tenure review. I am particularly pleased that evaluations from students taking course offerings for our new doctoral program and a newly re-structured course, N599, have received exceptionally positive feedback. Encouraging educational scholarship among these students has led the way to three different collaborative papers that are underway from course work with students— "Nurses with Disabilities: Professional Positions After Academia," "Cultural Competence in Health Care," and "Violations of Nursing Norms," which have been drafted for submission to peer-reviewed journals.

In summary, I have been able to excel at teaching even though this is my first academic teaching position. As noted by my director in my midpoint evaluation, "Since her arrival to Drexel University, Dr. Waite has consistently received above average to excellent teaching evaluations. This perhaps is remarkable since she came to Drexel with so little teaching experience." Similar comments were noted by the midpoint tenure review committee. For the first 4 years of my appointment (2003–2007), I taught exclusively in the undergraduate programs. A central goal was for me to gain more experience teaching at the graduate level and earn a doctoral teaching appointment. Since 2007, I was conferred a doctoral appointment by the associate dean of research. Currently, I teach across the doctoral, master's, and undergraduate programs. Evaluations in teaching across levels as reported in my 2008 evaluation by my director indicated, "Dr. Waite's teaching evaluation is above average overall and she got very good evaluations for her doctoral course. I do also note that Dr. Waite seems to excel at online teaching— not something I see every day."

In closing, my goal is to immerse students in a learning environment that is motivating, enlightening, and rigorous, where students freely practice, ask questions, think critically, and develop a desire and enthusiasm for life-long learning. I believe my teaching philosophy and my teaching style exudes my passion for the profession and my commitment to teaching nursing students that which is necessary for them to emerge as competent professional nurses who know both how to learn on their own and how to work with diverse groups of citizens. I am confident that these students will not only make a positive contribution to the profession, but more importantly, make positive contributions to the lives of individuals, families, and communities they serve.

### Teaching Critique

*Dr. Waite's section about teaching is well thought out and guides the reader with headings and transitional statements. She uses an eclectic philosophical base and identifies three main themes. She clearly explains each of them and how she enacts them. She is also pragmatic and describes what she does as a teacher and how it fits with her philosophy and goals.*

## RESEARCH AND SCHOLARSHIP

My research and scholarship began 6 years ago. It was most fortuitous that I was awarded a post-doctoral research fellowship (2005–2007), which has been a significant and positive influence on my research and scholarship activities. Principles that have guided my work are embedded in theoretical underpinnings found in the fields of anthropology, psychology, sociology, nursing, and human ecology. My work emphasizes three areas that have overlapping themes that complement each other within (and at the nexus of) mental health promotion, cultural competence, and behavioral research. I discuss each of these areas below.

## Educational Research

*Professional development among ethnic minority nursing students.* Successfully engaging students to embrace research while they are pursuing academic success in an undergraduate associate's degree in nursing (ADN) program is critical to their professional development. To help increase students' success in meeting these endeavors the Community College of Philadelphia, College of Nursing and Drexel University, College of Nursing and Health Professions have collaborated on a NIH grant to examine how structured didactic and research experiential activities influence student academic and professional outcomes. As the co-investigator (25% effort) on this $623,987, 3-year NIH grant, *Research Models for Change: Bridges to Baccalaureate,* I have had the opportunity to work in varied facets with participants. *Research Models for Change* afforded the research team a way to support students' reach beyond what is and what they know to forming alliances with exceptional nurse researchers who were from varied cultural backgrounds.

Students in this research took part in 15 months of academic experience and research-based experiential training in 2 phases (Level One and Level Two) to foster student interest in research and increase preparedness to transition to a 4-year institution of higher education. Participants obtained experiences in both primary care and health promotion wellness nursing centers, and acquired competencies to perform the technical skills required to participate in basic research. Participants were afforded significant research experiences in community and academic settings to work closely with experienced faculty on funded and dissertation projects including myself, the co-investigator of this project. CCP students were also given unique opportunities to relate course work in nursing, informatics, and research in nursing with delivery of comprehensive health care services to vulnerable populations in north and west Philadelphia. Importantly, these courses emphasize evidence-based practice, quality improvement approaches, and use of technology to facilitate problem solving. Students also obtained experience in scholarly writing (CV p. 14, "The lived experience of participating in research at a NNCC affiliated nurse managed center," *NNCC Update,* pp. 35–36) and professional presentations (CV p. 7, "Depression and the feminization of HIV and the silent epidemic in the US"; CV p. 10, "The intersection of obesity and depression").

Many of the participants in this research were: (1) the first in their families to attend higher education; (2) nontraditional students with most between 31 and 40 years of age; (3) African American followed by Hispanic and Asian populations; and (4) parents. While students were assessed for inclusion through a brief in-person interview and screened based on grade point average before taking part in this research, a central part of students' success in *Research Models for Change* was their readiness to take on added challenges of didactic, experiential, and research activities while already situated in an ADN program. Findings from this study indicated that readiness must be considered from informal and formal standpoints, as both had implications on students' ability to ascend toward their academic and professional goals as noted in our manuscript published in *Teaching and Learning in Nursing Education* (CV p. 4).

## Clinical Research

My community service, teaching, clinical experience, and education, particularly my post-doctoral studies, have provided me with the foundation to evolve as a clinical researcher. The focus of my clinical research has been

to gain a better understanding of mental health disparities among various populations, particularly African
Americans. By gaining an authentic and holistic view of
these issues, one is positioned to develop strategies that
can be developed to address inequities in states of mental health and well-being experienced by various population groups. My commitment to understanding more
about why and how target populations seek mental and
behavioral health services and the need to advocate for
mental health promotion will be discussed in the following paragraphs specifically related to (1) depression and
African American women, (2) health disparities that are
associated with undiagnosed and untreated trauma, and
(3) adult ADHD.

## Depression Research

I have a commitment to gaining a better understanding
about (1) how African American women articulate and
conceptualize depression, (2) African American wom-
en's health beliefs about depression, and (3) how African
American women manage depression in their daily lives.
Exploration of these factors is requisite to understanding treatment decisions pertaining to depression as well
as women's perceptions of vulnerability and social barriers related to treatment for depression. The *Diagnostic
and Statistical Manual of Mental Disorders*, fourth edi-
tion, text revision, tends to emphasize the universality
of depressive symptoms with modest attempts to identify
culture-related syndromes; however, gender and sociocul-
tural dimensions assist in shaping the psychological realities of African American women. Funding for research
was awarded through two competitive grants: an internal competitive grant through Drexel University and an
external competitive grant through Sigma Theta Tau, Nu

Eta Chapter. Concepts that were examined related to *what* depression means, health beliefs about depression, *why* enacting on addressing depression may occur, and *how* this plays out in their world and within the context of the lives of populations of African American women. Results from my scholarship in this area have led to several publications: *Journal of the American Psychiatric Nurses Association, Archives of Psychiatric Nursing, Archives of Psychiatric Nursing,* and the *Journal of Chi Eta Phi Sorority (JOCEPS)* and peer-reviewed presentations (CV, pp. 7–9).

Gaining a better understanding of authentic emic (subjective) perspectives using an anthropological explanatory model and a psychological health belief model is critical to inform communication about depression as well as its underlying cause(s). In collaboration with the Eleventh Street Family Health Center, a nursing health center known for its national model for care delivery by Innovative Care Models, the findings from these research studies afforded the researcher an opportunity to examine factors gleaned from the voices of women which in turn influenced how services were provided within the nurse-managed community health care center where participants received care for health and wellness needs. Consideration of qualitative data is requisite to improve patient-provider engagement. It is also critical for development of treatment and wellness activities that provide the best evidence for effective, appropriate, and culturally sensitive care to meet the needs of individuals affected by depression. Support groups at the Center were initiated and screening instruments, such as the Patient Health Questionnaire-9 and the Edinburgh Postnatal Depression Scale, have been used to track changes in symptom severity over time.

Findings from this research further identified the need for improved recognition and management of depression among African American women to mitigate morbidity and mortality for which they are disproportionately affected. For example, an area of interest that a collaborative team and I are exploring is associated behavioral and mental implications of depression among HIV-positive African American women using psychological and human ecology theoretical models. In collaboration with the Director of Psychiatry of Infectious Disease at 1427 Vine Streets, Drexel University, School of Medicine, we applied for an R 15 NIH grant which was not funded; however, plans are underway to reapply for a NIH grant.

Moreover, by conducting focus group research in the previously mentioned depression studies, an underlying concept was found to be a predominate theme—undiagnosed and untreated trauma among women participants. Similar findings continued to surface in the ongoing support groups started by the Eleventh Street Center. I am fortunate to have formed relationships through this work that led the Director of the Eleventh Street Family Health Services of Drexel University to invite me to be the Research Scientist at the Center.

## Trauma Research

As a Co-Primary Investigator on a competitive Barra Foundation grant, I have the opportunity to work with an eminent public health administrator, Dr. Patricia Gerrity, to examine integrative care for traumatic life experiences. Research has shown that both childhood maltreatment and psychological trauma in adulthood have been associated with increased vulnerability to psychiatric illness and more medical illness. While anecdotal and select group understanding of trauma has been examined, our funded study will replicate the Adverse Childhood Events Study (ACES) for all adult patients who receive services at the Eleventh Street Center. Fundamental research questions will examine (1) how traumatic life experiences affect an individual's health outcomes and (2) how adults' ACE scores correlate with chronic health concerns (physical and mental). By identifying the predominant types of trauma experienced by patients, we will then be able to strategize with interdisciplinary members (e.g., licensed social workers, integrative healers, couple and family therapists, creative art therapists, patient stakeholders, and registered nurses) to determine the most useful culturally appropriate methods of delivering care that will benefit and promote the well-being of patients at the Center. This study is currently in progress.

## ADHD Research

Another important component of my research focuses on adult ADHD. I was afforded an opportunity to explore critical aspects of ADHD among ethnic minority populations through a competitive grant awarded by the American Nurses Foundation. There is a dearth of literature and research that encompasses gender and cultural concerns about ADHD, specifically among ethnic minority adults across developmental stages and in different contexts. Given the far-reaching adverse implications that disparities in diagnosis and treatment of ADHD has on the affected individuals, their families, and their communities, it is requisite that clinicians and researchers identify factors that contribute to service disparities. This study specifically examined these factors among college students. To disseminate findings from this study, five papers have been developed and sent to respected, peer-reviewed interdisciplinary and nursing journals; three have been accepted for publication (*Journal of Psychosocial and Mental Health Services, Issues in Mental Health Nursing,* and *Journal of Attention Disorders*) and two are under review (*Women*

*& Health* and *Archives of Psychiatric Nursing*). To expound further on findings from the aforementioned study, I was selected from a competitive group of faculty and received the Christian R. and Mary F. Lindback Foundation Award in June 2009. By using a descriptive, exploratory concurrent triangulation design that examined gender differences related to severity of ADHD symptoms, depressive symptoms, and risk behaviors, I have been able to glean specific information that will support the development of an intervention study among college populations.

I am also the Principal Investigator on a NIMH proposal that is under review. Examining ADHD in community-based primary health care with parents of children diagnosed with ADHD is critical given the high heritability of the disorder. Undiagnosed parents face a chronic, potentially debilitating disorder with ambiguous treatment trajectories. By using innovative models—Parental Help-Seeking Behavioral Model for ADHD and a Parental Stages of Change Model—and theoretical constructs that take into account not only individual but also cultural and contextual factors, findings from this study are expected to advance the knowledge of the facilitators and eliminate barriers to help-seeking among parents who screen >14 on the Adult ADHD Self-Report Screener. Study findings will also inform the design of ADHD service interventions for parents from diverse backgrounds.

Relationships formed during my post-doctoral studies have helped forge partnerships with experts in the field at the University of Pennsylvania, Adult ADHD Center. Through ongoing collaborations, we have developed a scholarly paper, I have been invited to serve on a professional advisory board for Attention Deficit Disorder Association, and I have been invited to several professional presentations. By combining my role as an academician and researcher, I am uniquely positioned to conduct clinically focused research that will have a direct impact on mental and behavioral health disparities in the community and educational setting.

## Mentorship and Research/Scholarly Activities

In accordance with my teaching philosophy (i.e., *sharing knowledge and responsibility for learning*), I have included student participation from diverse disciplines in almost every study that I have conducted. Student participants in *Research Models for Change* took part in my depression research. I mentored them while they were completing their associate's degree in nursing. Likewise, student participants (a master's student in public health and a graduate nursing student) worked with me in various roles on my ADHD research. They shared in four peer-reviewed manuscripts that were developed; one manuscript is published, one is in press, and two are under review. Most recently, I was funded through a collaborative project through the provost's office at Drexel University to mentor an undergraduate psychology research co-op student. She is a member of our research team who is actively working on our trauma grant. We have (1) co-presented our research at Drexel University, Research Co-Op Recognition Symposium, (2) been selected to present a paper at a national conference in November, and (3) developed a peer-reviewed manuscript entitled "Adverse childhood experiences and its impact on mental health outcomes: Risk reduction by frontline practitioners," which will be submitted to the *Journal of the American Psychiatric Nurses Association*. I also mentor students through their master's theses and doctoral dissertations. Importantly, these students seek my advisement on research activities from interdisciplinary sectors (e.g., Creative Arts, Psychology, Couple and Family Therapy, and Nursing). In spring of 2009, two students completed their graduate thesis/

dissertation and graduated. Currently, I am advising five doctoral students; I am the supervising professor for two of these students, co-supervising professor for one, and serve as a committee member for two students.

## Summation

Specific goals from my midpoint tenure review were to increase my scholarly productivity by publishing in peer-reviewed journals, to continue to seek funding for clinical research activities, and disseminate findings in peer-reviewed presentations. At my midpoint review I had 3 peer-reviewed manuscripts published; 1 peer-reviewed book chapter; 5 peer-reviewed paper presentations; and 6 peer-reviewed poster presentations. Since then I have developed 20 peer-reviewed manuscripts (7 data-based); 4 peer-reviewed book chapters/contributions; 27 peer-reviewed paper presentations (nationally and internationally); and 13 peer-reviewed poster presentations. In accordance to my midpoint and 2008 evaluation I have achieved additional goals—invited as a journal editorial board member for *Perspectives in Psychiatric Care* and invited by the board chair of the Attention Deficit Disorder Association (ADDA) to serve on ADDA's Professional Advisory Board. Moreover, engagement of doctoral students has increased across disciplines and collaborative interdisciplinary partnerships have also taken place.

### Research Critique

*Dr. Waite not only tells the reviewers about her research but she describes how it connects to her teaching philosophy. This connection of themes ties things neatly together and shows how she is living her professional "passion." Dr. Waite breaks her research down into categories and provides a nice concise description of what the research is about.*

## SERVICE TO THE COMMUNITY/PROFESSION/ COLLEGE/UNIVERSITY

Service, another important area of my personal statement, has been guided by my authentic desire to be a good citizen within the community, my profession, and the college/university. Each will be addressed briefly in the following section.

### Service to the Community

Service that I have been able to provide to the larger community has been very rewarding. Through continued partnerships with churches, schools, and community mental health organizations, I have been able to share my knowledge and skills to help motivate and inform students' academic pursuits in general and specifically about the nursing profession. Engaging students in high school has also taught me the importance of connecting with students early on in their educational experience. Students are excited about the prospect of what lies ahead regarding their professional ambitions. While this is commendable, many students often lack an understanding of what nursing is about or the rigor that is involved to be successful. This can also be challenging, as many students are first-generation members of their families attending higher education. However, mentorship can help students develop as responsible citizens and individuals who are in pursuit of academic success. My service to churches has also been satisfying. Through educating and screening underserved populations for basic medical and mental health conditions, I am able to glean perspectives and concerns that are prominent from a grass-roots standpoint. Collaboration with larger community organizations (e.g., member of the Board of Directors for the Mental Health Association Southeastern Pennsylvania) provides an opportunity to ensure that innovative mental health education, advocacy programs, and mental health services are developed, maintained, and promoted in a culturally competent manner.

## Service to the Profession

My professional service is varied and expansive. My leadership role and collaborative partnerships have led to being on professional editorial boards, invited as a reviewer on several well established journals, and asked to review professional books and book chapters. Additionally, I am on the Board for the International Society for Psychiatric Nurses and take an active part in many other professional societies that the led way to being awarded the Trailblazer Award in 2007. In accordance with a central concept relevant to my work, mental health promotion within nurse managed primary health care centers, I have been honored to be Chair of the National Nursing Centers Consortium (NNCC) Mental Health Task Force for the past 3 years. My national service to the NNCC has afforded me opportunities for networking and for the development of collegial relationships that have led to collaborative partnerships on presentations and to initiatives that have influenced titling of psychiatric mental health advanced practice nurses (APNs) by the ANCC. A significant initiative is also currently underway that can change practice provisions for psychiatric APNs in Philadelphia County. Lastly, my professional service is strongly influenced by my commitment to the mentorship of students, supporting other nurse colleagues, and practicing, providing education about, and conducting research in a culturally competent fashion. I have been privileged to serve as a mentor for the National Coalition of Ethnic Minority Nurses Association for the past 3 years. Several manuscripts and presentations have developed from mentored relationships. Earlier this year, I was also awarded the Diversity Award based on my cultural competence development initiatives within the profession from the International Society for Psychiatric Nurses. I was also nominated and won the Excellence in Mentorship Award from Nursing Spectrum through nominations of my colleagues and mentees.

## Service to the College and University

Service to the college and university is also a significant part of my professional life. This encompasses committee membership on a university and college level and chairing committees on the college level. In addition to being elected to the Faculty Senate, I have served on the Provost's Committee on Faculty Diversity, Faculty Recruitment Committee and am serving on the Advisory Committee for University Offices of Multicultural Programs and the Institute for Women's Health and Leadership, Research Advisory Committee. For the past 4 years I have provided research-related service to the university as a CNHP judge on Research Day. Within the college, I serve on numerous committees and currently take leadership roles as Chair of the Tenure Track Doctoral Nursing Search Committee, Chair of the Emergency Protocol Committee, and serve as Vice-Chair of the Student Affairs Committee.

Student engagement is also a critical aspect of my college/university service. Through activity for 2 years on a HRSA grant ($836, 301), *Diversifying Nursing Care Delivery in Urban Healthcare*, I have served as the diversity coordinator. This grant aimed to increase nursing education opportunities for individuals from disadvantaged backgrounds including racial and ethnic minorities in order to provide a more diverse nursing workforce to meet society's needs. The grant focuses on pre-entry preparation, retention, and student scholarship/stipends. Two groups of students were targeted: high school seniors and transfer students at Drexel University, College of Nursing and Health Professions (CNHP) who were taking their first nursing course. As the diversity coordinator I took part in (1) providing workshops, (2) reviewing psychiatric mental health nursing content, (3) supporting with retention, (4) recruiting students from targeted high schools, and (5) serving as the liaison to the Undergraduate Nursing Diversity Organization (UNDO). In 2004, I started UNDO at Drexel University. Its mission is to promote cultural awareness, sensitivity, and support for all students in the undergraduate nursing program; create an open forum where students can discuss issues, concerns, and experiences within the undergraduate nursing program; and promote the development of skills needed to be responsible, accountable members of the nursing profession who respect the differences and similarities between people. Central to its goal is to work and build a campus community that empowers students and fosters diversity, academic excellence, equity, and cultural pluralism; also, to increase the matriculation, retention, and graduation rates of diverse student populations. As the advisor of this organization since its inception, I continue to be in awe of student initiatives for UNDO (e.g., taking part in community service activities, volunteer tutoring for middle school students, and fund raisers for external community groups in need of clothes and toiletry items). Through this student engagement, I am humbled and honored to have positively shaped the personal and professional lives of these students.

In summary, service to my profession, the community, and the university/college have excelled. My professional service has been substantive nationally and regionally through (1) review of professional journals both nursing and interdisciplinary, (2) book and chapter reviews, (3) mentoring in national organizations, (4) serving on a professional advisory committee and boards, and (5) active membership and participation in professional organizations. My community service has also been significant, especially through the presentations of health-oriented programs through community-based organizations. I have considerable university and college service. In accordance to my 2008 evaluation, my director commented, "Dr. Waite gives well-above-average service to the doctoral program. I have on occasion to call on Dr. Waite for extra service to the doctoral program and she is always receptive and performs at a high level."

### Service Critique

*Dr. Waite displays her vast service to all aspects that are considered for continuous tenure to the institution. She uses headers effectively and supports her statements with quotes and evidence in her appendix. Her vast service demonstrates investment to her students, the underserved communities which she affects, the educational institution, and to her career.*

## FUTURE GOALS

In this section, I will highlight my goals for the next 3 to 5 years for teaching, scholarship/research, and service—the trilogy of academe.

## Teaching

My ongoing quest to improve my teaching effectiveness is a process marked by failures as well as successes, and I do my best to learn from both outcomes. In light of this, I strive to maintain an honest, open mind and a spirit of humility in a process of continual evaluation. Teaching is such a rich and complex activity that opportunities for improving it abound. My efforts to improve my teaching have focused on (1) effective listening, (2) active learning, (3) respecting community, (4) increasing diversity, (5) effective student engagement for in-person and online classes, and (6) teaching across educational levels within the nursing programs at Drexel University. Teaching is one of the few professions that allows a person to influence a large group of people and to play a significant role in the cultivation of their knowledge and growth. Given that teaching is both a craft and a journey, my goals for the coming years are to further refine my teaching techniques to provide a stimulating learning environment for students, with the expectation that students not only acquire solid nursing knowledge, but also become culturally competent practitioners and acquire life-long active learning techniques. Specifically, I plan to:

1. Persist with idea sharing among colleagues regarding approaches to teaching, seeking out and using faculty development resources that target teaching effectiveness, and using frequent self-reflection.
2. Continue to enhance the incorporation of technology to enhance the student learning process for in-person and online classes.
3. Gain international experience with teaching in another country.
4. Incorporate an international perspective in my course requirements.

5. Continuously assess and advance my teaching strategies (in-class and online) in a manner that cultivates cultural sensitivity and higher-order thinking in students who are very diverse in their background, motivation, and learning styles.

## Scholarship/Research

My research and scholarship are influenced by wanting to produce best-practice and evidence-based knowledge and practice for health care workers and consumers in the context of the major, emerging mental impairments of the 21st century. My research and scholarship are contextualized by the convergence of diminishing health care resources, managed care, mental health disparities, and cultural diversification of consumers coping with multiple, chronic illnesses. Although I have gained significant experience and have contributed to extant literature and research, my goal is to continue to contribute new intellectual insights and positively impact the practice of the nursing profession in the areas of mental health promotion and behavioral research that take into account culture and context for individuals and families affected by ADHD, depression, and psychological trauma. To accomplish these goals I plan to:

1. Build upon my current research and apply for new funding to expand my work on ADHD once I have completed my currently funded grant. After completion of my active study, I will disseminate my work targeting interdisciplinary journals. Findings from this study should increase the breadth and depth of my inquiry about ADHD that will lead to the development of an intervention in collaboration with my colleagues (e.g., Adult ADHD Center at the University of Pennsylvania).

2. Strengthen international collaborations on publications, research, and presentations regarding ADHD (e.g., Dr. Julia Rucklidge at the University of Canterbury in New Zealand and Dr. Philip Asherson, from London's Maudsley Hospital).

3. Use findings from a current study underway examining trauma to seek funding to examine the efficacy and effectiveness of integrative care offered at the Eleventh Street Center for patients affected by traumatic events.

4. Strengthen interdisciplinary collaboration for research that examines mental and behavioral health indicators for HIV-positive African American women.

5. Continue to mentor future researchers through Drexel University doctoral programs and through serving on interdisciplinary dissertation and thesis committees.

6. Continue to publish scholarship and research findings in peer-reviewed journals and present nationally and internationally on best evidence for mental health promotion and behavioral indicators that enhance health and wellness for populations studied. I currently have several manuscript drafts that I will be publishing with students.

## Service

Service has been and continues to be an important and fundamental part of being a citizen and faculty member. I will continue my current professional, community, and university/college service and will seek to enhance my role in key areas as noted in the following. I have benefited as much from my service experience as have those individuals and groups to whom I have provided the service. This to me is the essence of service. As I move forward I plan to:

1. Increase my leadership roles in professional organizations.

2. Seek an associate editor or editor position on a national journal.
3. Continue to strengthen my networks with community groups.
4. Seek a leadership role on a university committee.

As I continue in my professional development, I know I still have to learn as much about myself as I can. I must constantly evaluate and re-evaluate my own beliefs, attitudes, values; my way of thinking about the specific material being examined and taught; my interpretation of the facts gathered; my assessment of the ideas and information to which I have been exposed; and my new level of knowledge, which is constantly being enhanced. Teaching is indisputably about sharing—sharing what I provide to my students while inviting them to share their knowledge and experiences with me. Ultimately, through my style of teaching, my dynamic approach, and my enthusiasm for my work, I hope to help students realize that self-empowerment is necessary for them to take responsibility for the content and quality of their own education. The reality is that the skills they will gain and the knowledge they will hopefully learn from their time at Drexel University will be transferred from the university setting to a series of real-world encounters that will amplify their life chances and their capacity to flourish within our society. I have only just begun my professional academic career and Drexel has provided a fruitful environment to advance my teaching skills, to participate in valuable scholarship/research, and to share my expertise with local communities. It is an honor to work at Drexel University and call it my professional home.

## SUMMARY

Writing a personal statement is the cornerstone of reflective practice in showcasing one's teaching, research and scholarship, and service-related activities. This exemplar is one approach to organizing a personal statement for a tenured position at a research intensive university. The critiques of each major section are intended to serve as teaching points. Be strategic in your thinking; engage the reader; use positive, assertive language; claim the significance and coherency of your contributions; and know the politics at your institution. In the end, you will make your case for being awarded tenure through telling your story as you reflect on this very important journey.

# References

Aiken, L. H., Clarke, S. P., Cheung, R. B., Sloane, D. M., & Silber, J. H. (2003). Education levels of hospital nurses and surgical patient mortality. *Journal of the American Medical Association, 290*, 1617–1623.

Alteen, A. M., Didham, P., & Stratton, C. (2009). Reflecting, refueling, and reframing: A 10-year retrospective model for faculty development and its implications for nursing scholarship. *The Journal of Continuing Education in Nursing, 40*(6), 267–272.

American Association of Colleges of Nursing. (2010). *Faculty shortage.* Retrieved from http://www.aacn.nche.edu/Media/Factsheets/facultyshortage.htm

American Nurses Association. (2008). BSN in ten. *American Nurse Today, 3*(11). Retrieved from http://www.americannursetoday.com/article.aspx?id=5272&fid=5244

American Nurses Credentialing Center. (2011). *ANCC Magnet Recognition Program®.* Retrieved from http://www.nursecredentialing.org/FunctionalCategory/FAQ/DEO-FAQ.aspx

American Psychology Association. (2009). *Publication Manual.* Washington, DC: APA Publications.

Appling, S. E., Naumann, P. L., & Berk, R. A. (2001). Using a faculty evaluation triad to achieve evidence-based teaching. *Nursing Health Care Perspective, 22*(5), 247–51.

Benner, P. (1984). *From novice to expert: Excellence and power in clinical nursing practice* (pp. 13–34). Menlo Park, CA: Addison-Wesley.

Billings, D., & Kowalski, K. (2008). Developing your career as a nurse educator: The professional portfolio. *The Journal of Continuing Education in Nursing, 39*(12), 532–533.

Boyer, E. L. (1990). *Scholarship reconsidered: Priorities of the professorate.* Princeton, NJ: Princeton University Press.

Carnegie Foundation for the Advancement of Teaching Basic Classifications of Schools of Higher Education in the U.S. (2010). Retrieved from http://classifications.carnegiefoundation.org/lookup_listings/standard.php

Casey, D. C., & Egan, D. (2010). The use of professional portfolios and profiles for career enhancement, *British Journal of Community Nursing, 15*(11), 547–552.

Children's Hospital of Philadelphia. (2011). *A Magnet institution.* Retrieved from http://www.chop.edu/service/nursing/a-magnet-institution.html

Corry, M. & Timmins, F. (2009). The use of teaching portfolios to promote excellence and scholarship in nurse education. *Nurse Education in Practice, 9*, 388–392.

Dictionary.com. (2011). Retrieved from http://dictionary.reference.com/browse/scholarship

Drexel University. (2011). *Mission statement.* Retrieved from http://www.drexel.edu/about/mission.aspx

Driessen, E., Van Tartwijk, J., & Van Der Vleuten, C. (2007). Portfolios in medical education: Why do they meet with mixed success? A systematic review. *Medical Education, 41*, 1224–1233.

Fahrenfort, M. (1987). Woman emancipation by health education: An impossible goal? *Woman Education and Counseling, 10*(87), 25–37.

Francis Marion University. (2011). Francis Marion University Handbook.

Freire, P. (1970). *Pedagogy of the oppressed.* New York: The Continuum International.

Freire, P. (1992). *The pedagogy of hope.* New York: The Continuum International.

Freire, P. (1998). *Teachers as cultural workers: Letters to those who dare teach.* Boulder, CO: Westview Press.

Glasgow, M. E. S. (2009). Functioning effectively within the institutional environment and academic community. In R. A. Wittmann-Price & M. Godshall (Eds.), *Certified Nurse Educator (CNE) review manual* (pp. 213–231). New York: Springer Publishing.

Grossman, S. C., & Valiga, T. M. (2005). *The new leadership challenge: Creating the future of nursing.* Philadelphia: F. A. Davis.

Institute of Medicine. (2010). *The future of nursing: Leading change, advancing health.* Retrieved from http://www.iom.edu/Reports/2010/The-Future-of-Nursing-Leading-Change-Advancing-Health.aspx

Javinen, A., & Kohenen, V. (1995). Promoting professional development in higher education through portfolio development. *Assessment and Evaluation in Higher Education, 20*(1), 25–36.

LaRocco, S. A. (2006). Who will teach the nurses? *Academic Online.* Retrieved from http://www.aaup.org/AAUP/pubsres/academe/2006/MJ/feat/laro.htm

Lewallen, L. P., & Kohlenberg, E. (2011). Preparing the nurse scientist for academia and industry. *Nursing Education Perspectives, 32*(1), 22–25.

Luk, A. M., Yukawa, M., & Emery, H. (2009). Disseminating best practices for the educator's portfolio. *Medical Education, 43,* 497–498.

Martsolf, D. S., Dieckman, B. C., Cartechine, K. A., Starr, P. J., Wolf, L. E., & Anaya, E. R. (1999). Peer review of teaching: Instituting a program in a college of nursing. *Journal of Nursing Education, 38*(7), 326–332.

McColgan, K., & Blackwood, B. (2009). A systematic review protocol on the use of teaching portfolios for educators in further and higher education. *Journal of Advanced Nursing, 65*(12), 2500–2507.

McCready, T. (2007). Portfolios and the assessment of competence in nursing: A literature review. *International Journal of Nursing Studies, 44,* 143–151.

Melland, H. I., & Volden, C. M. (1996). Teaching portfolios for faculty evaluation. *Nurse Educator, 21*(2), 35–38.

Morin, K. (2006). Faculty Q & A. *Journal of Nursing Education, 45*(7), 245–246.

Murray, J. P. (1994). Portfolios: Classroom moments frozen in time. *Academic Leader, 10*(10), 1–3.

National Institutes of Health. (2011). *Glossary and acronyms.* Retrieved from http://grants.nih.gov/grants/glossary.htm

National League for Nursing. (2005). *Competency 8—Function within the Educational Environment.* Retrieved from http://www.nln.org/facultydevelopment/pdf/corecompetencies.pdf

Nibert, M. (n.d.). *Boyer's Model of Scholarship*. Retrieved from http://www.webs1.uidaho.edu/mkyte/ui_strategic_plan_ implementation/resources/Boyer%20module%20Pacific%20 Crest%20recd%209.4.06.pdf

Oermann, M. (1999). Developing a teaching portfolio. *Journal of Professional Nursing, 15*(4), 224–228.

Oermann, M. (2002). Developing a professional portfolio in nursing. *Orthopaedic Nursing, 21*(2), 73–78.

O'Mara, L., Carpio, B., Mallette, C., Down, W., & Brown, B. (2000). Developing a teaching portfolio in nursing education: A reflection. *Nurse Educator, 25*(3), 125–130.

Peterson, C. A., & Sandholtz, J. H. (2005). New faculty development: Scholarship of teaching and learning opportunities. *Journal of Physical Therapy Education, 19*(3), 23–29.

Reece, S. M. Pearce, C. W., Melillo, K. D., & Beaudry, M. (2001). The faculty portfolio: Documenting the scholarship of teaching. *Journal of Professional Nursing, 17*(4), 180–186.

Romyn, D. M. (2000). Emancipatory pedagogy in nursing education: A dialectic analysis. *Canadian Journal of Nursing Research, 32*, 119–138.

Seldin, P., & Miller J. E. (2009). *The academic portfolio*. San Francisco: Jossey-Bass.

Suplee, P., & Gardner, M. (2009). Fostering a smooth transition to the faculty role. *The Journal of Continuing Education in Nursing, 40*(11), 514–520.

Sweitzer, H. F. (2003). Getting off to a good start: Faculty development in professional programs. *The Journal of Continuing Education in Nursing, 34*(6), 263–272.

Urbach, F. (1992). Developing a teaching portfolio. *College Teaching, 40*(2), 71–74.

Wilcox, J. & Brown, R. (2002). *Accreditation of prior and experiential learning—A student guide*. Retrieved from http://www.materials.ac.uk/resources/library/apelstudents.pdf

Wittmann-Price, R. A., Waite, R., & Woda, D. H. (2011). The role of the educator (pp. 161–176). In H. M. Dreher & M. E. S. Glasgow (Eds.), *Role development for doctoral advanced nursing practice*. New York: Springer Publishing.

# Appendix

## Contributors' Biographies

---

## RHONDA BROGDON, MSN, MBA, DNP, RN

Rhonda Brogdon is an assistant professor at Francis Marion University in Florence, SC. She has been a medical-surgical nurse for 16 years. She received her BSN degree from Clemson University in Clemson, SC, in 1994; her MSN degree from the University of Phoenix in Phoenix, AZ, in 2004; her MBA degree from Webster University located in Myrtle Beach, SC, in 2001; and her Doctorate in Nursing Practice (DNP) from Duquesne University located in Pittsburgh, PA, in 2010. Rhonda has served as mentor and preceptor for 12 years in bedside nursing and was consistently evaluated as a "role model" nurse for 10 years while working in acute care by her nurse manager. In academia, she has mentored and precepted faculty to their roles in course instruction for approximately 6 years.

Rhonda began working in academia as a part-time clinical nursing instructor at the Medical University of South Carolina/Francis Marion University Satellite in 2001. During that time, she had instructed all levels of nursing students in the clinical setting. Rhonda currently teaches Health Assessment and Nursing Research to pre-licensure students and Nursing Research to RN-BSN students.

Rhonda is co-editor of an article entitled, "Encouraging a Holistic Decision-Making Process in Healthcare." She has served as an external abstract peer reviewer for the Fourth Annual Healthcare Informatics Symposium presented by the Center for Biomedical Informatics at the Children's Hospital of Philadelphia, and she is currently working on publication of her DNP capstone project.

## FRANCES H. CORNELIUS, MSN, PhD, RN-BC, CNE

Frances H. Cornelius is Associate Clinical Professor, Chair of the MSN Advanced Practice Role Department and Coordinator of Informatics Projects at Drexel University, College of Nursing and Health Professions. Fran has taught nursing since 1991 at several schools of nursing. She taught community health at Madonna University (Livonia, MI), Oakland (MI) University, University of Pittsburgh, and Holy Family College (Philadelphia). Fran taught Adult Health and Gerontology at Widener University School of Nursing until 1997 when she began teaching at Drexel. In 2003, she was a Fellow at the Biomedical Library of Medicine. She is a certified nurse informaticist and has been the recipient of several grants. She has collaborated on the development of mobile applications as Coordinator of Informatics Projects including Patient Assessment and Care Plan Development (PACPD) tool, which is a PDA tool with a Web-based companion, and Gerontology Reasoning Informatics Programs (the GRIP project). She is the Co-Editor of Cornelius/Gallagher-Gordon, PDA Connections (Lippincott-Williams-Wilkins), an innovative textbook designed to teach health care professionals how to use mobile devices for "point-of-care" access of information. She has written 6 book chapters and has published 19 journal articles on her work. She has been invited to delivered 26 presentations and has delivered more than 50 peer-reviewed presentations mostly in the United States, but also in Spain, Canada, and Korea. She is a member of STTI, the American Informatics Association, the American Nursing Informatics Association, the International Institute of Informatics and Systemics (IIIS), NANDA, ANA, and the PSNA.

## JEANA N. DUNN, BSN, RN

Jeana N. Dunn attended the Academy for Technology and Academics during her junior and senior years of high school in order to attend a specialized class to gain experience in the nursing field. Getting a jump-start on her nursing career, she received her Certified Nursing Assistant (CNA certificate) in 2007. After graduating as Valedictorian of her Aynor High School class in 2007, she attended a community college until she was accepted into the Francis Marion University's (FMU) in Florence, SC, Baccalaureate of Nursing Program. While a student there, she served as a member of the FMU Nursing Curriculum Committee and Nursing Honor Society and the FMU Honors Student Association, and was a President's List member from 2007–2010; she was elected to membership of Phi Kappa Phi Honor Society and Cambridge Who's Who Registry from 2008–2010, and was recipient of the FMU Palmetto Gold Scholarship for 2009–2010. Following graduation from FMU in December of 2010, she was hired as an RN on a Maternal Child Health Services/Labor and Delivery unit. Jeana looks forward to future opportunities to continue her education so she can become a nurse educator.

## ROSEMARY FLISZAR, PhD, RN, CNE

Rosemary Fliszar is an Assistant Professor and MSN Coordinator in the nursing program at Kutztown University in Kutztown, PA. Rosemary has been a nurse for 40 years with extensive experience in Adult-Health/ Critical Care nursing and nursing education. She received her diploma from Lankenau Hospital School of Nursing in Philadelphia, PA, her BS in Nursing from Cedar Crest College in Allentown, PA, and her MSN in Adult Health/ Gerontology from DeSales University in Center Valley, PA. Rosemary completed her PhD at Duquesne University, Pittsburgh, PA (2003). Her dissertation explored the culture care practices of elderly Puerto Ricans living in a mid-size urban community. Rosemary has taught in diploma, ADN, BSN, RN-BSN, and MSN programs. She is a chapter contributor of several books, has published in professional journals, has presented at local, regional, national, and international conferences, and is a peer reviewer for *The Journal of Nursing Scholarship*. In addition to her study for her dissertation, Rosemary's areas of research include examining student needs in an online program and other areas of nursing education, as well as contributing as a qualitative researcher for a study conducted by Dr. Ruth A. Wittmann-Price examining women's choices in birth delivery methods.

## KAREN K. GITTINGS, DNP, RN, CCRN

Karen K. Gittings is an Assistant Professor of Nursing at Francis Marion University. Karen received her diploma in nursing from The Washington Hospital School of Nursing and her BSN from the University of Maryland, Baltimore County campus. She received her MSN with specialization in nursing education and her DNP from Duquesne University in Pittsburgh, PA.

Karen has extensive experience in critical care nursing and has been a certified critical-care registered nurse (CCRN) since 1991. Her areas of teaching expertise are medical-surgical nursing, critical care, and cardiac nursing. She has taught both junior- and senior-level undergraduate, baccalaureate nursing students in the classroom and clinical settings. Karen has a publication in *Nursing2011* on nurses' perceptions of how their body art is interpreted. She has also presented nationally on intravenous education through simulation.

Karen is a member of Sigma Theta Tau International Honor Society of Nursing and Phi Kappa Phi. She is currently the Vice President of the Francis Marion University Department of Nursing Honor Society and past President of the Pee Dee Area Chapter of the American Association of Critical Care Nurses. She is a recipient of multiple Outstanding Faculty Caring Teacher Awards at Francis Marion University and the South Carolina Palmetto Gold Award (2005).

## ROBERTA WAITE, EdD, APRN, CNS-BC

Roberta Waite is a tenured Associate Professor and serves as the Assistant Dean of Academic Integration and Evaluation of Community Programs, Drexel University (Philadelphia). She is a graduate of Widener University (BSN) and the University of Pennsylvania (MSN). She also earned a Doctorate in Higher Education Administration-Leadership from Widener University and completed a 2-year postdoctoral research fellowship (T32) at the

Center for Health Disparities Research at the University of Pennsylvania.

Her scholarly work focuses on help-seeking behaviors and treatment engagement with particular interest in depression, adult ADHD, and trauma and adversity among ethnic minority populations. Her research trajectory focuses on understanding these experiences, their affects on health behaviors, and responses in adult populations. She continues to explore behavioral research outcomes that promote early identification and recovery for individuals and families so that services and resources are provided to manage, mitigate, and avoid adverse health outcomes. Motivating and sustaining health behavior changes in minority populations and applying these findings to the practice settings are critical.

She has served on the Foundation Board of Directors for the International Society for Psychiatric Mental Health Nurses, Southeastern Area Pennsylvania Black Nurses Association, National Attention Deficit Disorder Association, Mental Health America of Southeastern Pennsylvania, and the Black Women's Health Alliance. She is also on the editorial board for *Perspectives in Psychiatric Care*.

# Index

========================================= *Other FAST FACTS Books*

**Fast Facts for the NEW NURSE PRACTITIONER:** *What You Really Need to Know in a Nutshell*, Aktan

**Fast Facts for the ER NURSE:** *Emergency Room Orientation in a Nutshell*, Buettner

**Fast Facts for the CLINICAL NURSE MANAGER:** *Managing a Changing Workplace in a Nutshell*, Fry

**Fast Facts for EVIDENCE-BASED PRACTICE:** *Implementing EBP in a Nutshell*, Godshall

**Fast Facts for the FAITH COMMUNITY NURSE:** *Implementing FCN/Parish Nursing in a Nutshell*, Hickman

**Fast Facts for the CARDIAC SURGERY NURSE:** *Everything You Need to Know in a Nutshell*, Hodge

**Fast Facts for the WOUND CARE NURSE:** *Practical Wound Management in a Nutshell*, Kifer

**Fast Facts for the CRITICAL CARE NURSE:** *Critical Care Nursing in a Nutshell*, Landrum

**Fast Facts for the TRAVEL NURSE:** *Travel Nursing in a Nutshell*, Landrum

**Fast Facts for the SCHOOL NURSE:** *School Nursing in a Nutshell*, Loschiavo

**Fast Facts for the MEDICAL OFFICE NURSE:** *What You Really Need to Know in a Nutshell*, Richmeier

**Fast Facts for CAREER SUCCESS IN NURSING:** *Making the Most of Mentoring in a Nutshell*, Vance

**Fast Facts for DEVELOPING A NURSING ACADEMIC PORTFOLIO:** *What You Really Need to Know in a Nutshell*, Wittmann-Price

**Fast Facts for the CLINICAL NURSING INSTRUCTOR:** *Clinical Teaching in a Nutshell*, Zabat Kan, Stabler-Haas

========================================= *Forthcoming*

**Fast Facts for the PSYCHIATRIC NURSE:** *Psychiatric Mental Health Nursing in a Nutshell*, Masters

**Fast Facts for DEMENTIA CARE:** *What Nurses Need to Know in a Nutshell*, Miller

**Fast Facts about the GYNECOLOGICAL EXAM for NURSE PRACTITIONERS:** *Conducting the GYN Exam in a Nutshell*, Secor and Fantasia

**Fast Facts for the CLASSROOM NURSING INSTRUCTOR:** *Classroom Teaching in a Nutshell*, Yoder-Wise, Kowalski

Visit www.springerpub.com to order.